AROMATHERAPY FOR LIFE

Reference Guide for 55 Common Essential Oils, Carrier Oils, and Hundreds of Recipes for Healthier Living

Jennifer C Spivey

Free Gifts For You!

Visit the Site Below to Download 3 Free E-Books!

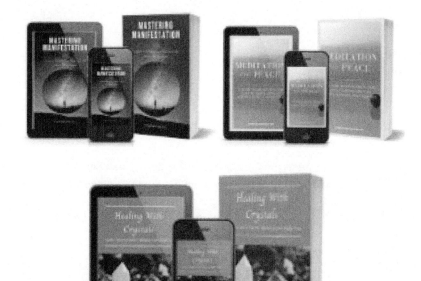

https://holistichealershop.com/free/

DEDICATION

This book is dedicated to my Aunt Sandi. Her support, belief in my abilities and encouragement has been a huge influence in my life.

Contents

Introduction

"The first wealth is health." -Ralph Waldo Emerson

I was first introduced to aromatherapy when I began a career in massage therapy and have been obsessed ever since. The fantastic feedback from my clients was immense. Not only did they benefit from aromatherapy, but I did as well by exposure to the essential oils while I was massaging my clients.

When I first started learning more about aromatherapy and essential oils, I was a little overwhelmed by how many oils there were, how to use safely, dilution guidelines, how to blend, etc. That began my quest to create a book referencing commonly used essential oils, carrier oils, easy to follow charts, the wonderful benefits of essential oils and carrier oils and lastly, fun as well as beneficial DIY recipes.

I have tried to simplify the process of learning about aromatherapy and essential oils without overwhelming you with too much information. You will see quite a few charts throughout the book that are great for reference. Whether you are new to aromatherapy and essential oils or a veteran, my hope is that you will love and benefit from these precious oils as I have.

PART I: ESSENTIAL OILS & CARRIER OILS

"Health is the greatest possession. Contentment is the greatest treasure. Confidence is the greatest friend. Non-being is the greatest joy." -Lao Tzu

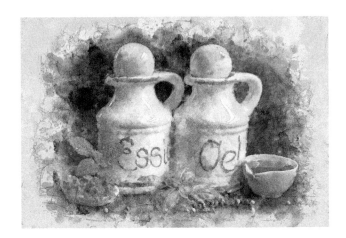

- What is Aromatherapy?

- Essential Oil Safety

- 55 Common Essential Oils

- Essential Oil Blending Basics

- Carrier Oil Properties

CHAPTER 1: AROMATHERAPY & ESSENTIAL OILS

"It is no measure of health to be well adjusted to a profoundly sick society." –
Jiddu Krishnamurti

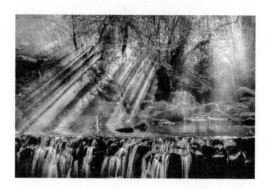

The use of aromatherapy and essential oils dates back over 10,0000 years to India. The Indians have used essential oils in their practice of ayurvedic medicine. The Egyptians, dating back to 4500 BC, were experts in the art of aromatherapy, especially with their embalming process.

Aromatherapy, also called essential oil therapy, is the use of plant derived essential oils for therapeutic purposes. Aromatherapy can be used in baths, massage lubricants, candles, diffusers, and much more!

We do not smell with the nose; we smell with our brains. With the sense of smell (olfaction), aromatherapy can be used to relax or stimulate the nervous system.

Concentrated essences of aromatic plants are known as **essential oils**. There are hundreds of pure essential oils available, however we will be discussing 55 commonly used essential oils throughout this book. These essences are 75 to 100 times stronger than the dried version of the plant. This strength is the primary reason for dilution before its use. Since essential oils are so concentrated, only small amounts, or drops are used.

Essential oils are extracted from botanicals by several methods, most commonly steam distillation. These precious oils are regarded as the soul of the plant by aromatherapists. Essential oils can be obtained from many parts of the plants. The following are examples:

• Flowers (e.g., jasmine, lavender)

• Fruits (e.g., lemon, bergamont)

• Grasses (e.g., lemongrass, citronella)

• Leaves (e.g., peppermint, eucalyptus)

• Roots (e.g., ginger, vetiver)

• Seeds (e.g., black pepper, fennel)

• Tree Blossoms (e.g., clary sage, ylang-ylang)

• Woods and Resins (e.g., frankincense, sandalwood)

In this book you will learn how aromatherapy can benefit your health, treat aches and pains, clean naturally, prepare skin care products, and much more! Hope you enjoy!

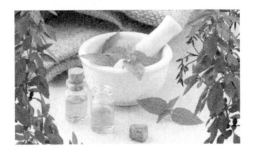

CHAPTER 2: ESSENTIAL OIL SAFETY

"It is health that is real wealth and not pieces of gold and silver." - Mohandas Gandhi

Being that essential oils are so concentrated; safety is important when dealing with essential oils. Essential oils are powerful so please treat them as such. Below are several guidelines when using on your skin, babies, children, and pregnant or lactating mothers.

Using Essential Oils on Skin:

• In most cases, essential oils should not be used undiluted on the skin.

• Undiluted use on the skin could cause an allergic reaction or irritation.

• As a general rule for adults, essential oils should be diluted in a carrier oil such as almond oil in a 1-5% dilution. (1-5 drops of essential oil per teaspoon of carrier oil)

Using Essential Oils on Babies and Children:

• Essential oils should never be used undiluted on skin or given internally.

• Dilution will be less for babies and children than for adults (See Dilution Chart)

• Certain oils considered "hot" could cause damage to the skin.

• In most cases lavender, orange, frankincense, lemon, and chamomile are considered safe for diluted use on children but do a skin test first. Also, check with your doctor.

• Peppermint, rosemary, eucalyptus, and wintergreen should never be used around babies or children. These herbs contain menthol and 1,8-cineole. These compounds can slow breathing or even stop it completely especially with young children or children with respiratory problems.

Using Essential Oils During Pregnancy or Nursing:

• Certain oils should be avoided during pregnancy or nursing due to their chemical makeup. This includes diffusing as well.

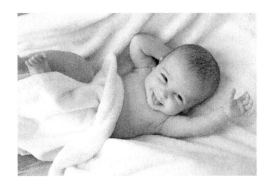

Safe Dilution Guidelines

Diluting essential oils is done by adding a drop or more of the essential oil with a carrier oil such as almond oil or jojoba oil. Not only does it provide a good medium for the oil to absorb into the skin, but also spreads the oil over a larger portion of your skin for better results.

Essential oils, being *lipophilic* (fat loving), require a fatty material not only to dilute it but also to suspend it. These materials are referred to as carrier oils because they help to carry the essential oil. Carrier and essential oils also compliment one another's effects; the skin easily absorbs them.

Knowing how to dilute properly will help you use essential oils safely. Even oils with safety concerns can be used if properly diluted.

Dilution is important for two reasons: one being skin reactions such as irritation, sensitivity, and phototoxicity and the other is systemic toxicity.

Below are some general guidelines for safely diluting essential oils. It is recommended that you use the lowest dilution possible for safety reasons. ***Please Note: These are only general guidelines. There may be other factors which would override these guidelines.***

Average Healthy Adult:

• 2% Dilution – 2 Drops essential oil per teaspoon of carrier oil: 12 Drops per ounce

Children 2-6 Years Old:

• 0.25% Dilution – 1 Drop essential oil per 4 teaspoons of carrier oil. (Hydrosol and Herbs are a good choice for this age group and should be considered before essential oils.)

Over 6 Years of Age:

• 1% Dilution – 1 Drop essential oil per teaspoon of carrier oil: 6 Drops per ounce. (Also recommended for pregnant women, elderly adults, those with skin sensitivities, compromised immune systems, or other serious health issues.)

CONVERSIONS	1% DILUTION	2% DILUTION
2 Tbsp = 1 fl. oz = 30 ml = 6 tsp	1 oz = 30 ml = 600 drops of oil	1 oz = 30 ml = 600 drops of oil
1 tsp = 5ml = 100 drops	1% of 600 drops is 6	2% of 600 drops is 12
1 tsp of carrier oil + 1 drop of essential oil = 1%	Add 6 drops of essential oil for 1 oz of carrier oil or finished product.	Add 12 drops of essential oil for 1 oz of carrier oil or finished product.

Please Note: If you are unsure about using aromatherapy on yourself or a child due to health concerns, please reach out to a qualified aromatherapist.

Essential Oils to Avoid with Children

Listed below are essential oils which should be avoided with children by diffusion, topically, or both. Some essential oils have several different chemotypes of species, some that are safe for children and some that are not.

If you want to inhale essential oils not safe for kids, I suggest you use a personal inhaler instead of a diffuser. You can still reap the benefits and not affect your children.

If you do decide to diffuse essential oils not safe for children, be sure the diffuser is not in a room that your children will be in. After diffusing, give the room at least an hour to air out before allowing your children to enter.

When applying topically under clothing, allow 15-30 minutes before getting close to your children. This should give the essential oil enough time to evaporate so the aroma is virtually undetected when you are around your children.

When applying topically to exposed skin, give yourself about 30 minutes before getting close to your children. Higher dilutions of essential oils for example, a muscle blend, using Peppermint and Eucalyptus at a 20% dilution may take longer to evaporate (up to an hour), but a 2% dilution of the same might be safe after 15 minutes.

• **Anise/Aniseed** *Pimpinella anisum*– avoid using with children under 5

• **Anise (Star)** *Illicium verum*– avoid using with children under 5

• **Basil (lemon)** *Ocimum x citriodorum*– avoid topical use on children under 2

• **Benzoin** *Styrax benzoin, Styrax paralleloneurus, Styrax tonkinensis* –

avoid topical use on children under 2

• **Birch (sweet)** *Betula lenta*– avoid using with children

• **Black Seed** *Nigella sativa*– avoid topical use on children under 2

• **Cajuput** *Melaleuca cajuputi, Melaleuca leucadendron*– avoid using with children under 6

• **Cardamon** *Elettaria cardamomum*– avoid using with children under 6

• **Cassia** *Cinnamomum cassia, Cinnamomum aromaticum*– avoid topical use on children under 2

• **Chaste Tree** *Vitex agnus castus*– avoid using with prepubertal children

• **Clove Bud, Clove Leaf, Clove Stem** *Syzygium, Eugenia caryophyllata, Eugenia aromatica*- avoid topical use on children under 2

• **Cornmint** *Mentha arvensis, Mentha canadensis*– avoid using with children under 6

• **Eucalyptus** *Eucalyptus camaldulensis, Eucalyptus globulus, Eucalyptus maidenii, Eucalyptus plenissima, Eucalyptus kochii, Eucalyptus polybractea, Eucalyptus radiata, Eucalyptus Australiana, Eucalyptus phellandra, Eucalyptus smithii* – avoid using with children under 10

• **Fennel(bitter), Fennel(sweet)** *Foeniculum vulgare*– avoid using with children under 5

• **Galangal (lesser)** *Alpiniaofficinarum, Languas officinarum*– avoid using with children under 6

• **Garlic** *Allium sativum*– avoid topical use on children under 2

• **Ginger Lily** *Hedychium coronarium*- avoid topical use on children under 2

• **Ho Leaf/Ravintsara** *Cinnamomum camphora* (cineole chemotype)–

avoid using with children under 6

• **Hyssop** *Hyssopus officinalis (pinocamphone chemotype)*–avoid using with children under 2

• **Laurel Leaf/Bay Laurel** *Laurus nobilis* – avoid topical use on children under 2; avoid all routes for children under age 6

• **Lemon Leaf/Lemon Petitgrain** *Citrus x limon, Citrus limonum* – avoid topical use on children under 2

• **Lemongrass** *Cymbopogon flexuosus, Andropogon flexuosus, Cymbopogon citratus, Andropogon citratus*- avoid topical use on children under 2

• **Marjoram (Spanish)** *Thymus mastichina*– avoid using (all routes) with children under 6

• **Massoia** *Cryptocarya massoy, Cryptocaria massoia, Massoia aromatica* –avoid using with children under 2

• **May Chang** *Litsea cubeba, Litsea citrata, Laura cubeba*– avoid topical use with children under 2

• **Melissa/Lemon Balm** *Melissa officinalis*- avoid topical use with children under 2

• **Myrtle (red)** *Myrtus communis*– avoid using with children under 6

• **Myrtle (aniseed***) Backhousiaanisata*– avoid using with children under 5

• **Myrtle (honey)** *Melaleuca teretifolia*– avoid topical use on children under 2

• **Myrtle (lemon)/***Sweet Verbena Backhousiacitriodora*– avoid topical use on children under 2

• **Niaouli (cineole chemotype)** *Melaleuca quinquinervia* –avoid using on children under 6

• **Oakmoss** *Evernia prunastri*– avoid topical use on children under 2

• **Opopanax Commiphoraguidottii**- avoid topical use on children under 2

• **Oregano** *Origanum onites, Origanum smyrnaeum, Origanum vulgare, Origanum compactum, Origanum hirtum, Thymbra capitata, Thymus capitatus, Coridothymus capitatus, Satureeja capitata* – avoid topical use onchildren under 2

• **Peppermint** *Mentha x Piperita* – avoid using with children under 6

• **Peru Balsam** *Myroxylon balsamum, Myroxylon pereira, Myroxylon peruiferum, Myrospermum pereirae, Toluifera pereirae*- avoid topical use on children under 2

• **Rambiazana Helichrysum** *gymnocephalum*- avoid using with children under 6

• **Rosemary (1,8-cineole chemotype)** *Rosmarinus officinalis*- avoid using with children under 10

• **Saffron** *Crocus sativus*– avoid topical use on children under 2

• **Sage (Greek)** *Salvia fruiticosa, Salvia triloba* –avoid using with children under 6

• **Sage (White)** *Salvia apiana*– avoid using (all routes) with children under 6

• **Sage (Wild Mountain)** *Hemizygia petiolata*– avoid topical use on children under 2

• **Sanna** *Hedychium spicatum*– avoid using (all routes) with children under 6

• **Saro** *Cinnamosma fragrans*– avoid using (all routes) with children under 6

• **Savory** *Satureia hortensis, Satureia montana*– avoid topical use on children under 2

• **Styrax** *Liquidambar orientalis, Liquidambar styraciflua*– avoid topical use on children under 2

• **Tea Leaf/Black Tea** *Camellia sinensis, Thea sinensis*– avoid topical use on children under 2

• **Tea Tree (lemon scented)** *Leptospermum petersonii, Leptospermum citratum, Leptospermum liversidgei*- avoid topical use on children under 2

• **Treemoss** *Pseudevernia furfuracea* –avoid topical use on children under 2

• **Tuberose** *Polianthes tuberosa*– avoid topical use on children under 2

• **Turpentine** *Pinus ayacahuite, Pinus caribaea, Pinus contorta, Pinus elliottii, Pinus halepensis, Pinus insularus, Pinus kesiya, Pinus merkusii, Pinus palustris, Pinus pinaster, Pinus radiata, Pinus roxburghii, Pinus tabulaeformis, Pinus teocote, Pinus yunnanensis*- avoid topical use on children under 2

• **Verbena (Lemon)** *Aloysia triphylla, Aloysia citriodora, Lippa citriodora, Lippa triphylla*- avoid topical use on children under 2

• **Wintergreen** *Gaultheria fragrantissima, Gaultheria procumbens* – avoid on children under age 10 due to methyl salicylate content

• **Ylang-Ylang** *Cananga odorata*– avoid topical use on children under 2

Essential Oils to Avoid While Pregnant or Nursing

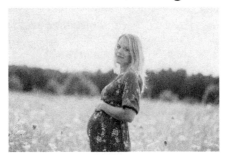

These essential oils have been determined to be unsafe for use during pregnancy and lactation, whether topical or by diffusion because their chemical makeup contains specific chemical constituents that should be avoided during pregnancy.

Aniseed (Pimpinella anisum)	May Chang
Anise, Star (Illicium verum)	Melissa
Araucaria (Neocallitropsis pancher)	Mugwort (common, camphor/thujone CT)
Artemisia (Artemisia vestita)	Mugwort (common, chrysanthenyl acetate CT)
Atractylis (Atractylylodes lancea)	Myrrh (Commiphora myrrha)
Basil (lemon)	Myrtle (aniseed)
Birch sweet (Betula lenta)	Myrtle (honey)
Black Seed (Nigella sativa)	Myrtle (lemon)
Buchu (Agathosma betulina, Agathosma crenulata)	Oregano (Origanum onites, Origanum smyrnaeum, Origanum vulgare, etc.)
Calamint (Calamintha nepeta)	Parsley leaf

Carrot Seed (Daucus carota)	Parsley seed
Cassia (Cinnamomum cassia)	Pennyroyal (Mentha pulegium)
Chaste Tree (Vitex ugnus castus)	Rue (Ruta graveolens)
Cinnamon Bark (Cinnamomum verum)	Sage, Dalmatian (Salvia officinalis)
Cypress, blue (Callitris intratopica)	Sage, Spanish (Salvia lavandulaefolia)
Dill Seed, Indian (Anethus sowa)	Tansy (Tanacetum vulgare)
Fennel, bitter and sweet (Foeniculum vulgare)	Tea Tree (lemon scented)
Feverfew (Tanacetum parthenium)	Thuja (Thuja occidentalis)
Genipi (Artemisia genepi)	Thyme (lemon)
Hibawood (Thujopsis dolobratta)	Verbena (lemon)
Ho Leaf (Cinnamomum camphora)	Western Red Cedar (Thuja plicata)
Hyssop (pinocamphone CT)	Wintergreen (Gaultheria procumbens)
Lanyana (Artemisia afra)	Wormwood (all chemotypes)
Lavender, (Spanish) (Lavandula stoechas)	Yarrow (green)
Lemon Balm, Australian (Eucalyptus staigeriana)	Zeodary
Lemongrass	

Essential Oil Safety with Pets

We cannot forget about our furry friends when it comes to aromatherapy and essential oils! Although there are safe essential oils for pets, you should never intentionally or unintentionally let your animals ingest these oils or apply directly to their skin undiluted. I would recommend checking out Plant Therapy's blog for more detailed information on using essential oils on or around your pets. The following is a just a general reference guide on safety precautions for your pets.

If you are interested in trying aromatherapy with your pets, please talk to your vet beforehand to ensure that you are not exposing your animals to toxic oils and be sure to study proper handling methods. Below is a list of essential oils that are potentially toxic to **Dogs: Tea Tree, Cinnamon, Clove, Thyme, Garlic, Sweet Birch, Juniper, and Yarrow**

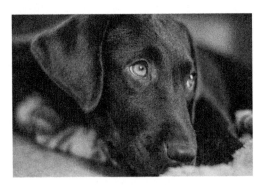

For Cats, follow these simple tips to enjoy your oils while simultaneously keeping your kitty safe!

• Diffuse in a well-ventilated room blocked off from your cat.

• Never diffuse in an enclosed room with your cat trapped inside.

• Store your essential oils somewhere your cat cannot reach them to prevent accidental contact and/or ingestion.

• If applying diluted oils to yourself topically, avoid your cat for at least an hour. Do not pet them or let them lick you.

• Wash your hands thoroughly after working with oils.

• When using essential oils in cleaning products, do not allow your cat to walk on those surfaces until the oils have evaporated. Absorption through paws or ingestion during grooming will increase your cat's chance of poisoning.

• Using inhalers is the perfect way to enjoy your oils without putting any cats in harm's way!

Following these suggestions will help to minimize your cat's exposure to essential oils and therefore decrease the likelihood of any toxins building up in his or her body.

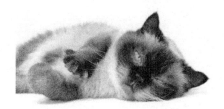

CHAPTER 3: 55 COMMON ESSENTIAL OILS

"The wish for healing has always been half of health."
-Lucius Annaeus Seneca

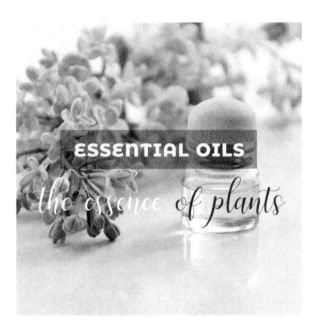

Amyris Essential Oil

Botanical Name: Amyris balsamifera

Country of Origin: Haiti

Extraction Method: Steam distilled

Plant Part: Wood

Strength of Aroma: Medium

Aromatic Scent: Amyris is dry, woodsy, peppery balsamic

Blends Well With: Cedarwood Atlas, Citronella, Cypress, Frankincense Carteri, Jasmine Absolute, Lavandin, Lemon, Mandarin, Rose Absolute, Sandalwood Australian, Orange Sweet

Amyris Essential Oil is wonderful for relaxation, particularly before sleep. Amyris is a thick, pale yellow essential oil steam distilled from the wood of a tree native to Haiti and other tropical climates. Amyris is also sometimes called West Indian Sandalwood or Torchwood; however, its properties are different, and it is not botanically related to true Sandalwood oil.

Balsam Fir Essential Oil

Botanical Name: Abies balsamea

Country of Origin: Canada

Extraction Method: Steam distilled

Plant Part: Needles

Strength of Aroma: Medium

Aromatic Scent: Distinctively woodsy

Blends Well With: Black Pepper, Citronella, Frankincense, Juniper Berry, Lavender, Lemon, Pine Scots, Spruce, Tea Tree.

With an uplifting yet soothing effect, Balsam Fir is an excellent oil for calming muscles and joints. When diffused or applied topically to the chest, this oil can help support a healthy respiratory system. Additionally, Balsam Fir is used by many for its emotional balancing effects.

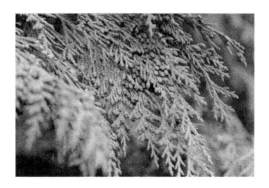

Balsam Fir

Bergamot Essential Oil (Bergapten Free)

Botanical Name: Citrus bergamia

Country of Origin: Italy, France, Guinea, Ivory Coast

Extraction Method: Cold Pressed

Plant Part: Fruit Peel-1 kg oil yield from: 200–250 kg of the rinds

Strength of Aroma: Medium

Aromatic Scent: Citrusy and fruity with a warm spicy floral quality

Blends Well With: Clary Sage, Cypress, Frankincense Carteri, Geranium, Grapefruit Pink, Jasmine, Mandarin, Orange Sweet, Patchouli, Black Pepper, Sandalwood Australian, Vetiver

Cautions: *Buy Bergapten Free Bergamot, which is safe for use in the sun. If not, you should not go out into the sun uncovered for 24 hours as it is highly phototoxic.*

Bergamot is a favorite amongst essential oil users for its aroma and therapeutic properties. Its scent is citrusy with a hint of floral making it unique and vibrant. This wonderful aroma is known for its ability to help boost the mind and ease your worries, especially during times of sadness and grief.

Bergamot is gentle for skin care and can assist with teenage skin problems and oily skin. It is also a favorite to add to massage blends to help reduce muscle tension and give relief from tightness caused by overexertion or achy muscles.

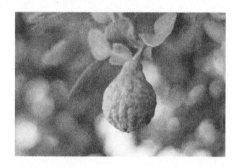

Bergamont

Black Pepper Essential Oil

Botanical Name: Piper nigrum

Country of Origin: India

Extraction Method: Steam Distilled

Plant Part: Fruit

Strength of Aroma: Medium

Aromatic Scent: Warm and fresh, dry-woody scent

Blends Well With: Bergamot, Copaiba Balsam, Cypress, Frankincense, Geranium, Juniper Berry, Rose Absolute, Sandalwood and Vetiver

The warm, mild aroma of Black Pepper will remind you of freshly ground peppercorns combined with a soft floral scent. Black Pepper is an excellent choice to help in reducing occasional discomfort after exercise or easing achy joints, menstrual pains and is antiseptic so it is great for the diffuser in cold and flu season.

Blue Cypress Essential Oil

Botanical Name: Callitris intratropica

Country of Origin: Australia

Extraction Method: Steam Distilled

Plant Part: Wood

Strength of Aroma: Weak

Aromatic Scent: Woody, balsamic, and fresh with subtle sweet notes.

Blends Well With: Black Pepper, Cedarwood Atlas, Cedarwood Virginian, Copaiba Balsam, Cypress, Helichrysum Italicum, Lavender, Lemon, Rose Absolute, Sandalwood

This pleasant blue oil is obtained by steam distilling the wood of this native Australian tree. The only other "blue" essential oils known in aromatherapy are obtained from flowers. Like most of the "blue" oils, Blue Cypress is a wonderful support for reddened, congested skin, can help keep minor skin breaks "clean", and can help with respiratory support. For emotional uses, it is known to be calming and soothing to a restless spirit.

Blue Tansy Essential Oil

Botanical Name: Tanacetum annuum

Country of Origin: Morocco

Extraction Method: Steam distillation of the fresh herb as soon as the first flower buds appear from mid-July through early September-1 kg oil yield from: 300–400 kg of the fresh herb

Plant Part: Aerial Parts

Strength of Aroma: Medium

Aromatic Scent: An herbaceous, sweet apple-like scent

Blends Well With: Clary Sage, Coriander Seed, Geranium, Juniper Berry, Lavender, Petitgrain, Rosalina, Rose Absolute, Spearmint, Turmeric CO2

Blue Tansy Oil is a magnificent oil that is cherished for its captivating scent and incredible clearing, calming properties. This oil has a rich blue hue and a sweet, clean scent. Blue Tansy provides relief for many people who suffer during high-pollen seasons, soothes troubled skin and is very calming emotionally.

Caraway Seed Essential Oil

Botanical Name: Carum Carvi

Country of Origin: Poland, Germany

Extraction Method: Supercritical Extraction

Plant Part: Seeds

Strength of Aroma: Medium

Aromatic Scent: Warm, rich, herbaceous aroma

Blends Well With: Black Pepper, Cardamom, Chamomile Roman, Frankincense Carteri, Sweet Orange

The main ingredients are Limonene, which is well-known for its stimulating and uplifting properties, and Carvone which helps with digestive issues. Caraway Seed CO2 has a warm, herbaceous scent.

This fragrance is very grounding and balancing to the senses but can also offer an energizing boost when you need to stay alert. The warm, rich scent is a favorite to use in perfumes or room spray to help mask odors found around the home or office.

Caraway Seed CO2 can be used for an energizing boost when feeling tired or lethargic. It is also a great support to a healthy digestive system and can be used to ease an occasional upset stomach. Use it to support a healthy respiratory system when seasonal threats occur and a healthy immune system all year long. Additionally, caraway seed essential oil is great for skin and hair care. It can be used to balance and cleanse the skin, especially individuals with oily or blemish-prone faces.

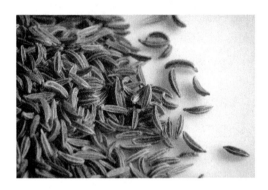

Caraway Seed

Cardamom Essential Oil

Botanical Name: Elettaria cardamomum

Country of Origin: Guatemala

Extraction Method: Steam Distilled

Plant Part: Seeds

Strength of Aroma: Medium

Aromatic Scent: Spicy aroma

Blends Well With: Balsam Fir, Frankincense Carteri, Lemon, Orange Sweet, Pine Scots

Cardamom Essential Oil has a sweet, spicy scent that will be familiar to those who are accustomed to Cardamom often used in Asian cuisine. This mighty oil is well-known for calming the respiratory and digestive system and can often provide relief to those who struggle on boats or lengthy car rides. As a traditional "warming" oil, Cardamom is stimulating and uplifting. It can assist with improving a low mood and is sometimes used to enhance romantic desire.

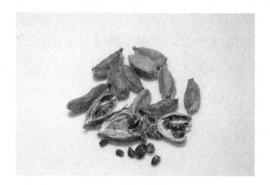

Cardamom

Cedarwood Atlas Essential Oil

Botanical Name: Cedrus atlantica

Country of Origin: Morocco/Algeria

Extraction Method: Steam Distilled-1 kg oil yield from: 30–50 kg of the dried wood chips

Plant Part: Wood

Strength of Aroma: Strong

Aromatic Scent: Dry woody aroma, slightly smoky, balsamic, and very subtle with a hint of spice

Blends Well With: Bergamot, Clary Sage, Cypress, Frankincense Carteri, Jasmine Absolute, Juniper Berry, Neroli, Pine Scots, Vetiver

Cedarwood Atlas has a rich, woody, slightly sweet and spicy aroma that reminds you of an antique cedar chest. This fantastic essential oil is known for its therapeutic properties throughout the oil world for its calming ability and help with staying focused and upbeat. Additionally, it can calm a racing mind so you can fall asleep.

You can also use this fantastic oil to help support a healthy respiratory system as well as a healthy, flake-free scalp. It is also great to use in a blend to keep those pesky bugs away.

Cedarwood Virginian Essential Oil

Botanical Name: Juniperus virginiana

Country of Origin: USA

Extraction Method: Steam Distilled

Plant Part: Wood

Strength of Aroma: Medium

Aromatic Scent: Fresh, clean, dry, woody and oily scent.

Blends Well With: Clary Sage, Copaiba Balsam, Cypress, Fir Needle, Frankincense Carteri, Lavender, Neroli, Patchouli, and Vetiver.

Cedarwood Virginian is a species of Juniper tree. It has an aroma similar to a freshly sharpened pencil, although it is more intricate. Cedarwood Virginian is popularly used in products formulated for men, due to its woodsy, outdoor scent. Its qualities are the same as atlas cedarwood above.

Chamomile German Essential Oil

Botanical Name: Matricaria chamomilla

Country of Origin: Egypt, Hungary, Nepal

Extraction Method: Steam Distilled-1 kg oil yield from: 300–500 kg of the fresh herb

Plant Part: Flowers

Strength of Aroma: Strong

Aromatic Scent: A strong, sweetish, warm, herbaceous odor

Blends Well With: Bergamot, Chamomile Roman, Clary Sage, Geranium, Jasmine Absolute, Lavender, Lemon, Neroli, Patchouli, Tea Tree

The powerful scent of Chamomile German is widely known for its calming properties and immensely helpful to children who have problems focusing. It is also an excellent soother of congested skin and can be used in blends to assist with seasonal pollen allergies. In addition, this versatile oil is great for skin healing and wounds, muscle spasms and cramps.

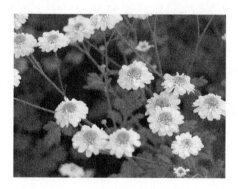

Chamomile

Chamomile Roman Essential Oil

Botanical Name: Chamaemelum nobile

Country of Origin: China, United Kingdom, USA, France

Extraction Method: Steam Distilled

Plant Part: Flowers-1 kg oil yield from: 80–100 kg of the fresh herb

Strength of Aroma: Strong

Aromatic Scent: Sweet, "green", herbaceous apple-like scent

Blends Well With: Bergamot, Chamomile German, Clary Sage, Geranium, Jasmine Absolute, Lavender, Lemon, Neroli, Patchouli, Tea Tree

The powerful, sweet scent is a favorite among essential oil users as a sleep aid for children and adults. It has a more calming effect than the German chamomile, so it is greatly beneficial for restless children. The soothing and gentle qualities of this oil also helps to ease tired muscles after strenuous exercise and aching joints.

Cinnamon Bark Essential Oil

Botanical Name: Cinnamomum verum

Country of Origin: Madagascar, Sri Lanka

Extraction Method: Steam Distilled

Plant Part: Bark

Strength of Aroma: Strong

Aromatic Scent: Woody, warm, sweet, spicy

Blends Well With: Clove Bud, Cypress, Ginger, Orange Sweet, Patchouli, Rosemary, Spearmint, Vanilla

Cinnamon bark creates a wonderful, warm, inviting atmosphere! This powerful essential oil not only creates a pleasant atmosphere but can also assist in keeping your home clean during seasonal illness. This marvelous oil can also help ease worry and reduce fatigue.

Citronella Essential Oil

Botanical Name: Cymbopogon winterianus

Country of Origin: Indonesia, China, India

Extraction Method: Steam Distilled

Plant Part: Leaves

Strength of Aroma: Medium

Aromatic Scent: Lemony citrus type scent, though it is much softer than actual Lemon with subtle wood tones

Blends Well With: Bergamot, Cedarwood, Geranium, Lavender, Lemon, Sweet Orange, and Pine Scots.

Citronella is often used in soaps and candles because of its refreshing scent. It can help to support a healthy respiratory system and aid in relaxation. Used topically, Citronella can make your time spent outdoors more pleasant and helps to keep the bugs away!

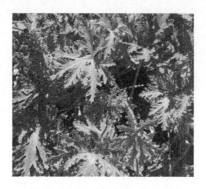

Citronella

Clary Sage Essential Oil

Botanical Name: Salvia sclarea

Country of Origin: France, Bulgaria, Crimea, England, Hungary

Extraction Method: Steam Distilled

Plant Part: Leaves and flowering tops-1 kg oil yield from: 100–150 kg of the herb

Strength of Aroma: Medium

Aromatic Scent: Earthy, fruity, and floral aroma that is both nutty and herbaceous

Blends Well With: Bergamot, Cedarwood, Chamomile German, Chamomile Roman, Geranium, Jasmine Absolute, Lavender, Neroli, Sweet Orange, Sandalwood

The wonderful aroma of Clary Sage is very earthy and has hints that are fruity, floral, nutty, and herbaceous. This very soothing aroma is the key blend that helps create an atmosphere that is balancing and calming when emotions are raging.

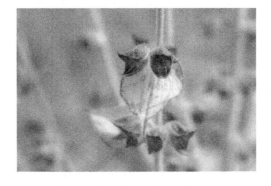

Clary Sage

Copaiba Oleoresin Essential Oil

Botanical Name: Copaifera officinalis

Country of Origin: El Salvador, Brazil

Extraction Method: Tree Tapping

Plant Part: Balsam

Strength of Aroma: Light

Aromatic Scent: Delicate, sweet, and smooth with a creamy-woody scent

Blends Well With: Pepper Black, Chamomile Roman, Cedarwood, Jasmine Absolute, Sandalwood, Vanilla CO2, Frankincense

Copaiba Oleoresin is a distinctive, gentle oil that is tree tapped from the Balsam of the Copaiba tree to produce a pure, undiluted oleoresin. This gentle, yet effective oil is known for its ability to alleviate sore muscles and joints. It is also a great warming addition to respiratory blends in cold and flu season and can relieve the occasional upset stomach.

Coriander Seed Essential Oil

Botanical Name: Coriandrum sativum

Country of Origin: Russia

Extraction Method: Steam Distillation

Plant Part: Seeds

Strength of Aroma: Medium

Aromatic Scent: Sweet, peppery, slightly fruity smell

Blends Well With: Bergamot, Clary Sage, Fir Needle, Grapefruit Pink, Lemon, Neroli, Orange Sweet, Petitgrain, Rose Absolute and Turmeric

Coriander Seed is a fragrant, exotic oil that has been used for thousands of years in Asian countries. It can stimulate the appetite and is excellent in relieving an upset stomach. It helps elevate mood, calms frazzled nerves, helps with mental focus and aids in relaxation before sleep. Coriander Seed Essential Oil is safe to use on congested or blemished skin.

Cypress Essential Oil

Botanical Name: Cupressus sempervirens

Country of Origin: Spain, France

Extraction Method: Steam Distilled

Plant Part: Leaves

Strength of Aroma: Medium

Aromatic Scent: Spicy, herbaceous, slightly woody evergreen aroma It is fresh and clean.

Blends Well With: Lavender, Tea Tree, Geranium, Cedarwood Atlas, Pine Scots, Orange Sweet, Sandalwood, Clary Sage, Juniper Berry, and Jasmine Absolute.

Cypress has a fresh, clean aroma that is herbaceous, spicy, with a slightly woody evergreen scent. This oil is a favorite because of its many therapeutic properties. Cypress can be used to support a healthy respiratory system and give emotional strength.

Cypress is ideal for supporting a healthy respiratory system all year long, especially during times of seasonal allergies. Additionally, Cypress is a great alternative to using eucalyptus. The uplifting aroma has a very soothing emotional quality that provides comfort during times of grief and sadness.

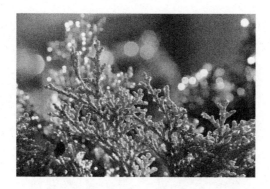

Cypress

Eucalyptus Globulus Essential Oil

Botanical Name: Eucalyptus globulus

Country of Origin: South-eastern Australia (native), Spain, Portugal, Morocco, Brazil, China

Extraction Method: Steam Distilled

Plant Part: Leaves

Strength of Aroma: Strong

Aromatic Scent: A very herbaceous scent with soft woody undertones

Blends Well With: Cedarwood, Chamomile, Cypress, Geranium, Ginger, Grapefruit Pink, Juniper, Lavender, Lemon, Marjoram, Peppermint, Pine, Rosemary, and Thyme

Cautions: *Do not apply to, or near, the face of infants or young children. Eucalyptus Globulus is one of the world's most familiar essential oils and is widely known to help with respiratory problems.*

Eucalyptus Globulus is also very effective as a support to aching muscles and joints from occasional overuse after a strenuous gym workout or with joint changes associated with the aging process. Eucalyptus can stimulate healthy circulation, bringing a feeling of warmth to the body. It can also be effective in stimulating mental focus.

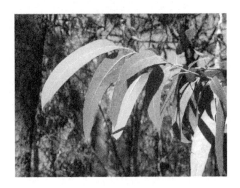

Eucalyptus

Eucalyptus Radiata Essential Oil

Botanical Name: Eucalyptus radiata

Country of Origin: Australia, South Africa

Extraction Method: Steam Distilled

Plant Part: Leaves

Strength of Aroma: Strong

Aromatic Scent: A crisp, clean, aroma with a hint of citrus and floral.

Blends Well With: Cedarwood, Coriander, Frankincense, Lavender, Pine, Rosemary, and Tea Tree

Cautions: *Do not apply to or near the face of infants or young children.*

Eucalyptus Radiata essential oil is often considered a milder Eucalyptus because it is slightly "smoother" than Eucalyptus Globulus and has a somewhat softer odor. Eucalyptus Radiata essential oil has a crisp, clean, aroma with a hint of citrus and floral. It has many of the same properties as Eucalyptus Globulus and they are often combined to help support a healthy respiratory system and to ease breathing.

Eucalyptus Radiata can help combat seasonal illnesses by helping you breathe easier. Use it in an aromatherapy diffuser to help clear the mind and keep you focused.

Fir Needle Essential Oil

Botanical Name: Abies sibirica

Country of Origin: Russia

Extraction Method: Steam Distilled

Plant Part: Needles / Twigs

Strength of Aroma: Medium

Aromatic Scent: A fresh, dry, resinous, piney aroma

Blends Well With: Chamomile Roman, Clary Sage, Coriander Seed, Cypress, Frankincense Carteri, Geranium, Juniper Berry, Black Pepper, Pine Scots, and Tea Tree.

The uplifting forest-fresh scent of Fir Needle is a wonderful respiratory support oil. Fir needle helps ease congested lungs associated with seasonal illness and seasonal pollen threats.

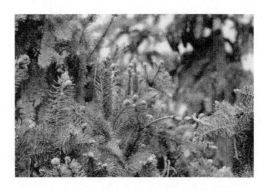

Fir Needle

Frankincense Carteri Essential Oil

Botanical Name: Boswellia carteri

Country of Origin: Somalia

Extraction Method: Hydro-distilled

Plant Part: Resin

Strength of Aroma: Medium

Aromatic Scent: Green, balsamic, with lemonwood

Blends Well With: Black Pepper, Cinnamon, Lime, Lemon, Cypress, Lavender, Geranium, Palmarosa, Patchouli, Rose, Sandalwood, Vetiver, Ylang Ylang

Frankincense Carteri essential oil is steam distilled from a Middle Eastern or African tree's gum resin. It has been used for thousands of years as a spiritual incense, folk medicine, and in cosmetics. In traditional Chinese Medicine, the gum resin is used for bruising, swelling, sores, and pain from traumatic injuries.

Frankincense Carteri can rejuvenate the look of mature skin and can be used in serums or creams for the face. It is also used as an immune system support.

Geranium Essential Oil

Botanical Name: Pelargonium x asperum

Country of Origin: South Africa, Madagascar, Réunion, Egypt, Morocco, China, India.

Extraction Method: Steam Distilled

Plant Part: Leaves-1 kg oil yield from: 500–700 kg of the fresh herb

Strength of Aroma: Strong

Aromatic Scent: Fresh, sweet, green, herbaceous scent

Blends Well With: Bergamot, Citronella, Lavender, Lemon, Palmarosa, Patchouli, Rose Absolute, Sandalwood

Geranium Egyptian is a wonderful skin-balancing oil that can improve the overall skin complexion. It is known for its beneficial effects on women's reproductive health and can be helpful in easing the tension associated with the stress of daily life. It is uplifting and gentle.

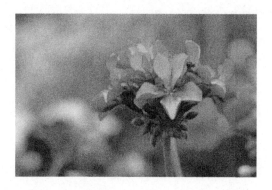

Geranium

Ginger Essential Oil

Botanical Name: Zingiber officinale

Country of Origin: Germany, Nigeria, Indonesia

Extraction Method: Supercritical CO2 Extraction

Plant Part: Rhizomes

Strength of Aroma: Strong

Aromatic Scent: Fresh, warm, and spicy/woody lemon scent

Blends Well With: Bergamot, Cedarwood Atlas, Clove Bud, Coriander Seed, Jasmine Absolute, May Chang, Sweet Orange, Petitgrain, Rose Absolute, Sandalwood, Turmeric

Traditionally used for its warming action, Ginger Root aids digestion, stimulates blood flow and helps relieve a queasy stomach and menstrual discomfort. When added to a carrier oil or lotion, it helps joint and muscle aches.

Grapefruit Pink Essential Oil

Botanical Name: Citrus x paradisi

Country of Origin: USA, South Africa

Extraction Method: Cold Pressed

Plant Part: Fruit Peel

Strength of Aroma: Light

Aromatic Scent: Sweet, juicy fresh citrus scent

Blends Well With: Citronella, Coriander Seed, Fir Needle, Geranium, Jasmine Absolute, Juniper Berry, Neroli, Petitgrain

Cautions*: Grapefruit oil can cause photosensitivity. Do not use more than 4% dilution as it can be phototoxic.*

Grapefruit Pink is great for mental fatigue and moodiness. It is also incredibly uplifting emotionally.

Helichrysum Italicum Essential Oil

Botanical Name: Helichrysum italicum

Country of Origin: France, Croatia, Bosnia

Extraction Method: Steam distillation of the fresh flowering herb in July and August

Plant Part: Flowering Plant-1 kg oil yield from: 1,100–1,400 kg of the fresh herb

Strength of Aroma: Medium

Aromatic Scent: Sweet, warm, herbal woody

Blends Well With: Bergamot, Pepper Black, Chamomile Roman, Clary Sage, Geranium Lavender, Lemon, Neroli, Palmarosa, Rose Absolute

True Helichrysum Italicum oil, also known as Immortelle, is grown only in a few spots around the world and is unsurpassed in its ability to rejuvenate the look of healthy, unblemished skin. Use it to reduce the appearance of scars and wrinkles, or other skin blemishes on the face or body.

Helichrysum Italicum is said to support the body through post-illness fatigue and convalescence, mainly through boosting normal immune function. Helichrysum Italicum oil also soothes deep emotional feelings and diffuses anger and destructive feelings. It is excellent for coughs and muscular aches and pains.

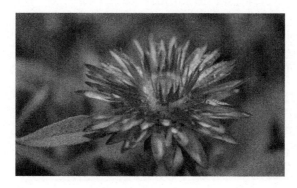

Helichrysum

Ho Wood Essential Oil

Botanical Name: Cinnamomum camphora

Country of Origin: China

Extraction Method: Steam distilled

Plant Part: Wood

Strength of Aroma: Medium

Aromatic Scent: Woody, floral and camphorous scent

Blends Well With: Bergamot, Cedarwood Atlas, Chamomile German, Chamomile Roman, Lavender, Lemon, Sandalwood

Ho Wood Oil is steam distilled from the bark and wood of the ho tree. This oil is extremely high in calming linalool and is excellent for promoting a peaceful and relaxing environment.

Ho Wood has a woody, floral, and camphorous scent. Its aroma and properties are very similar to Rosewood Oil, which as a threatened species, should be avoided. The camphor content in Ho Wood Oil results in a cooling feeling when used topically.

Jasmine Absolute Essential Oil

Botanical Name: Jasminum sambac

Country of Origin: India

Extraction Method: Solvent extraction

Plant Part: Flowers

Strength of Aroma: Strong

Aromatic Scent: Intense oily-fruity, waxy floral scent

Blends Well With: Bergamot, Clary Sage, Copaiba Balsam, Coriander Seed, Frankincense Carteri, Petitgrain, Rose Absolute, Sandalwood, Vanilla CO2, Vanilla Oleoresin

Jasmine Absolute is an incredible oil known for its distinctive, exotic floral aroma that is often used in perfumery. Its invigorating smell is known as an aphrodisiac that increases feelings of love and romance.

Additionally, it is enriching to the senses and helps to create a positive atmosphere. Other popular uses include helping to rejuvenate and refresh the skin when added to skincare products and soothing a sore throat.

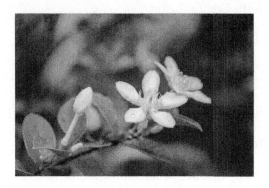

Jasmine

Juniper Berry Essential Oil

Botanical Name: Juniperus communis

Country of Origin: Bosnia-Herzegovina, Macedonia, Albania, Turkey, France, Italy, Hungary, England.

Extraction Method: Steam distilled

Plant Part: Berries-1 kg oil yield from: 100–300 kg of the dried ripe berries

Strength of Aroma: Medium

Aromatic Scent: Sharp green, woody conifer scent

Blends Well With: Bergamot, Clary Sage, Chamomile Roman, Coriander Seed, Cypress, Fir Needle, Frankincense, Grapefruit Pink, and Black Pepper.

Juniper Berry essential oil is an incredible oil with a very distinct scent and is a natural purifier. The sharp, green, woody, conifer scent can help soothe nervous tension and is ideal for meditation when added to a diffuser or personal inhaler.

When applied topically, it can produce a warming sensation making it a great choice to use on achy muscles after a strenuous workout. Use it after a long day on your feet in a foot bath for an invigorating treat to your feet.

Lavender Essential Oil

Botanical Name: Lavandula angustifolia

Country of Origin: Bulgaria, Spain, France, Greece

Extraction Method: Steam Distilled

Plant Part: Flowering Tops-1 kg oil yield from: 100–150 kg of the herb

Strength of Aroma: Medium

Aromatic Scent: Sweet, Dry, and Herbaceous-floral

Blends Well With: Bergamot, Cedarwood Virginian, Clary Sage, Geranium, Helichrysum, Lemon, Neroli, Patchouli, Rose Absolute, Sandalwood and Vetiver.

Lavender or Lavandula Angustifolia, is a full-bodied steam-distilled oil from the flowering tops of the Lavender plant. Known for its many uses, Lavender essential oil is world renowned as one of the world's most popular and versatile oils, and for good reason!

Lavender has an incredibly sweet, floral, herbal scent and is also highly valued for its many therapeutic properties. The smell of Lavender alone can help produce a calm, peaceful tranquil environment.

Diffuse Lavender essential oil into the air before bedtime to promote peaceful sleep or add Lavender to your favorite lotion or carrier oil to soothe the skin and help unwind your senses. It is also excellent for pains, burns, scrapes, and prevents scarring.

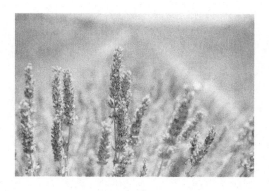

Lavender

Lemon Essential Oil

Botanical Name: Citrus x limon

Country of Origin: Italy, Spain, Israel, Argentina, USA

Extraction Method: Cold Pressed

Plant Part: Fruit Peel-1 kg oil yield from: 120–150 kg of the fresh rind

Strength of Aroma: Strong

Aromatic Scent: Fresh, zesty citrus scent

Blends Well With: Bergamot, Cedarwood Atlas, Citronella, Coriander Seed, Geranium, Lavender, Lime, Neroli, Palmarosa, Petitgrain, Sandalwood and Vetiver.

Lemon has a fresh, zesty citrus scent that is refreshing, energizing, and uplifting; this scent is invigorating to the senses and wonderful to smell. Hailing from Italy, Lemon Essential Oil has been used for centuries. This strong, but refreshing scented aroma is known to support healthy immune system, uplift and revitalize, and add a wonderful lemon scent to spray cleaners.

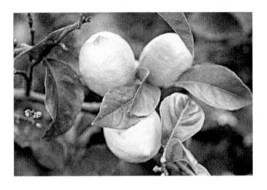

Lemon

Lemon Eucalyptus Essential Oil

Botanical Name: Corymbia citriodora

Country of Origin: Madagascar

Extraction Method: Steam Distilled

Plant Part: Leaves

Strength of Aroma: Medium

Aromatic Scent: Light, sweet lemony citronella-type scent

Blends Well With: Cedarwood Atlas, Citronella, Frankincense Carteri, Lavender, Lemon, Spearmint and Tea Tree.

Lemon Eucalyptus Essential Oil is calming to the spirit with its sweet lemony aroma. It's a wonderful air freshener and can help support a healthy respiratory system. Many people like to use Lemon Eucalyptus when spending time outdoors in the warmer months.

Cautions: *If pregnant or under a doctor's care, consult your physician.*

Lemongrass Essential Oil

Botanical Name: Cymbopogon flexuosus

Country of Origin: India

Extraction Method: Steam distilled

Plant Part: Leaves

Strength of Aroma: Strong

Aromatic Scent: Fresh-oily, lemony, tea-like scent

Blends Well With: Bergamont, Black Pepper, Cedarwood, Clary Sage, Coriander, Cypress, Fennel, Geranium, Ginger, Grapefruit, Lavender, Lemon, Marjoram, Orange, Palmarosa, Patchouli, Rosemary, Tea Tree, Thyme, Vetiver, and Ylang Ylang

Cautions: *To avoid the risk of various safety issues, use a maximum dilution of 0.7% for topical applications. Possible drug interactions.*

Lemongrass is known as being a helpful addition to outdoor sprays. It is refreshing and deodorizing when diffused, as well as being uplifting to the spirit. It can also be added to a carrier oil (well diluted) to boost circulation, bringing warmth to overused muscles and joints.

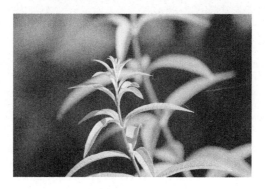

Lemongrass

Lime Essential Oil

Botanical Name: Citrus x aurantifolia

Country of Origin: Mexico

Extraction Method: Steam Distilled

Plant Part: Fruit Peel

Strength of Aroma: Medium

Aromatic Scent: Sweet green citrus scent

Blends Well With: Bergamot, Cardamom, Citronella, Clary Sage, Coriander Seed, Jasmine Absolute, Lavandin, Lavender, Lemon, Lemon Eucalyptus, Neroli, Sweet Orange, Petitgrain, Grapefruit Pink, Rose Absolute, Sandalwood, Vanilla Oleoresin.

Steam Distilled Lime Oil. unlike Cold Pressed Lime Oil, is not phototoxic. Therefore, you can feel free to add it to lotions, balms, and other body products without worrying about sun exposure.

Lime Oil has a beautifully clean, bright citrus scent with a hint of sweetness. The bright aroma of Lime makes a wonderful start to the day and can help clear and energize the mind. It can also help support a healthy immune system.

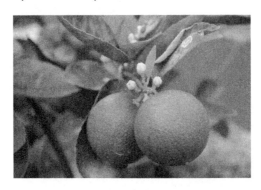

Lime

Mandarin Essential Oil

Botanical Name: Citrus reticulata

Country of Origin: Brazil, Italy, Israel, South Africa, Argentina,

Extraction Method: Cold Pressed

Plant Part: Fruit Peel-1 kg oil yield from: 100–150 kg of the fresh

fruit rinds

Strength of Aroma: Light

Aromatic Scent: Sweet, fresh, full-bodied citrus scent

Blends Well With: Cypress, Frankincense Carteri, Geranium, Lavender, Lemon, Lime, Neroli, Orange Sweet, Petitgrain, Rose absolute, Vanilla CO2

Because of its sweet, fresh scent, Mandarin is uplifting and can help soothe nervous tension and sadness when diffused.

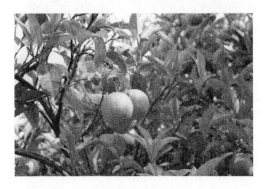

Mandarin

Marjoram Sweet Essential Oil

Botanical Name: Origanum majorana

Country of Origin: Egypt, Tunisia, Hungary, France

Extraction Method: Steam distilled

Plant Part: Flowers-1 kg oil yield from: 160–200 kg of the fresh herb

Strength of Aroma: Medium

Aromatic Scent: Fresh-medicinal, sweet, herbaceous scent

Blends Well With: Coriander Seed, Cypress, Dill Weed, Helichrysum italicum, Mandarin, Orange Sweet, Sandalwood and Tea Tree

Marjoram is calming and warming and can help encourage relaxation before sleep. When suffering from the symptoms of common seasonal illnesses, Marjoram can provide comfort.

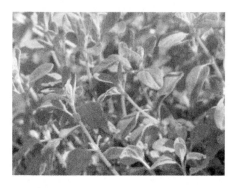

Marjoram

Neroli Essential Oil

Botanical Name: Citrus x aurantium

Country of Origin: Egypt, Morocco

Extraction Method: Steam distilled

Plant Part: Flowers

Strength of Aroma: Medium

Aromatic Scent: Beautiful orange blossom floral scent

Blends Well With: Bergamot, Geranium, Grapefruit Pink, Jasmine Absolute, Lavender, Lemon, Lime, Mandarin, Orange Sweet, Palmarosa, Petitgrain, Rose Absolute, Tangerine, Vanilla CO2 and Sandalwood

Neroli is the perfect essential oil for when you need a break from life. This delightful and vibrant floral essential oil comes from orange blossoms found in Egypt.

It is one of the most comforting and effective essential oils when dealing with grief, nervous tension, or exhaustion. Neroli is often used in skincare preparations to promote a healthy complexion.

Orange Sweet Essential Oil

Botanical Name: Citrus sinensis

Country of Origin: Brazil, USA, Greece, South America,

Extraction Method: Cold Pressed

Plant Part: Fruit Peel

Strength of Aroma: Medium

Aromatic Scent: Juicy-fresh, light citrus scent

Blends Well With: Bergamot, Coriander Seed, Fir Needle, Frankincense, Geranium, Jasmine Absolute, Lemon, Neroli and Vanilla

Orange Sweet is most known for its wonderful uplifting and calming scent. When diffused, it can help with nervous tension, sadness, and can also improve the aroma of a stale room. It can also help support normal function of the immune system.

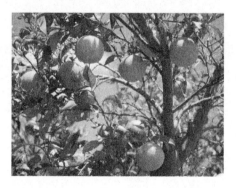

Sweet Orange

Palmarosa Essential Oil

Botanical Name: Cymbopogon martini

Country of Origin: India

Extraction Method: Steam distillation of the fresh or dried grass in April and May, and again September through December.

Plant Part: Leaves-1 kg oil yield from: 50–70 kg of the grass

Strength of Aroma: Medium

Aromatic Scent: Soft, Green & Rosy

Blends Well With: Bergamot, Cedarwood Virginian, Geranium, Lemon, Neroli, Patchouli, Petitgrain, Rose Absolute and Sandalwood

Palmarosa has a soft, sweet floral scent and is often diffused to freshen up and sanitize the air. It is also considered to be an excellent skin-balancing oil for all skin types, much like Neroli essential oil.

Palmarosa is a marvelous oil for supporting digestive health and is also viewed as helpful with uplifting and steadying the emotions. In addition, it is also a wonderful oil to use when seasonal illness strikes.

Patchouli Essential Oil

Botanical Name: Pogostemen cablin

Country of Origin: Indonesia (Sumatra), Malaysia, Seychelles, India, Madagascar, South China, Brazil

Extraction Method: Steam distilled

Plant Part: Leaves-1 kg oil yield from: 30–50 kg of the dried herb

Strength of Aroma: Medium

Aromatic Scent: Rich, Earthy, Woody, "Wine scent"

Blends Well With: Bergamot, Cedarwood Virginian, Geranium, Copaiba Balsam, Cypress, Lavender, Neroli, Orange Sweet, Palmarosa, Rose Absolute, Sandalwood, and Vetiver

Patchouli became famous during the 1960's in the United States as a favorite scent of young "hippies",but has been used as a scent in Asia for centuries. It is best known for its skin care applications.

When added to a carrier oil, it can help with the appearance of wrinkles, scars, and skin blemishes. It is also a wonderful addition to a man's deodorant formula. When diffused, Patchouli can help alleviate nervous tension and worry.

Peppermint Essential Oil

Botanical Name: Mentha x piperita

Country of Origin: India

Extraction Method: Steam Distilled

Plant Part: Leaves

Strength of Aroma: Strong

Aromatic Scent: Fresh, cool, grassy-minty scent

Blends Well With: Cypress, Eucalyptus, Geranium, Grapefruit, Juniper Berry, Lavender, Lemon, Marjoram, Rosemary, Tea Tree, and Oregano

Cautions: *Do not apply on or near the face of infants and children.*

Peppermint is a perennial herb that grows widely in Europe, North America, and Asia. This leafy plant grows close to the ground and produces smooth, dark green leaves with clusters of small pinkish lavender flowers.

Originated in India, Peppermint has been used for centuries for its revitalizing properties. Steam distilled from the leaves of the mint plant; Peppermint Essential Oil creates a strong aromatic scent that has a fresh, cool, grassy-minty smell. This scent is invigorating to the senses that promotes energy and alertness.

Peppermint is a refreshing and stimulating oil that is both soothing and enlightening. Peppermint Essential Oil has a cooling effect on the skin that is revitalizing and wonderful to the touch, due to its menthol content. It is great for joint and muscle pain and headaches.

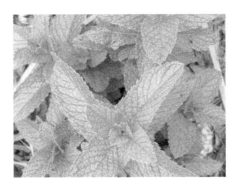

Peppermint

Petitgrain Essential Oil

Botanical Name: Citrus x aurantium

Country of Origin: Italy, Paraguay

Extraction Method: Steam Distilled

Plant Part: Leaves / Twigs

Strength of Aroma: Strong

Aromatic Scent: Bitter-sweet, woody floral scent

Blends Well With: Bergamot, Coriander Seed, Jasmine Absolute, Lemon, Lime, Mandarin, Neroli, Palmarosa, Grapefruit Pink

Petitgrain Essential Oil originated from Paraguay and is extracted using steam distillation from the leaves and twigs of the Seville bitter orange tree. This oil has a woodsy, fresh scent with a hint of floral. This wonderful aroma is a favorite for natural perfumery, comforting the mind when emotions are running wild, and is gentle and effective for skin care.

When added to body or room spray, the delightful scent of

Petitgrain can give the atmosphere not only a wonderful aroma but creates an environment that is uplifting and energizing.

During times of great emotional upheaval, Petitgrain is great to help balance emotions. A favorite for skin care, Petitgrain is gentle, yet effective to help with blemishes and oily skin.

Pine Scots Essential Oil

Botanical Name: Pinus sylvestris

Country of Origin: Austria, Hungary

Extraction Method: Steam Distilled

Plant Part: Leaves

Strength of Aroma: Strong

Aromatic Scent: Fresh, sweet-green woody scent

Blends Well With: Citronella, Clary sage, Frankincense, Grapefruit Pink

Pine Scots is particularly known for its ability to help support a healthy respiratory tract. When added to a carrier oil, it is warming and soothing to tired muscles and can help support circulation.

When added to cleaning products or potpourri, it brings the fresh scent of the forest into your home. In addition, Pine Scots is a great alternative to using eucalyptus. Massage onto your child's chest and/or diffuse to ease congestion, coughs, and sinusitis.

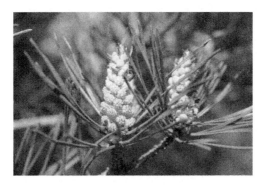

Pine Scots

Rosalina Essential Oil

Botanical Name: Melaleuca ericifolia

Country of Origin: Australia

Extraction Method: Steam Distilled

Plant Part: Leaves

Strength of Aroma: Medium

Aromatic Scent: Soft, lemony, medicinal, and floral scent

Blends Well With: Blue Tansy, Citronella, Cypress, Fir Needle, Geranium, Grapefruit Pink, Lavender, Lemon, Palmarosa, and Tea Tree.

Rosalina essential oil (also referred to as Lavender Tea Tree in Australia) has many of the same properties as Eucalyptus oil, yet it is gentler and safer. Rosalina oil is great for respiratory congestion common with seasonal pollen threats or wintertime illness.

Rose Absolute Essential Oil

Botanical Name: Rosa x centifolia

Country of Origin: Morocco

Extraction Method: Solvent extracted

Plant Part: Flowers

Strength of Aroma: Medium

Aromatic Scent: Sweet, green/waxy and floral

Blends Well With: Bergamot, Chamomile, Geranium, Helchrysum Italicum, Jasmine Absolute, Lemon, Neroli, Palmarosa, Patchouli, Petitgrain, Sandalwood Vetiver

Highly prized for its rich floral scent, Rose Absolute is also known for its calming properties, helping to soothe emotions and bring calm during fresh grief. It can promote relaxation before sleep when diffused or applied topically diluted in a carrier oil. It is extremely useful in skin rejuvenation, as Rose oil counteracts the visible signs of aging, reducing the appearance of wrinkles and helping smooth skin.

Rosemary Essential Oil

Botanical Name: Rosmarinus officinalis

Country of Origin: Tunisia

Extraction Method: Steam Distilled

Plant Part: Aerial Parts

Strength of Aroma: Strong

Aromatic Scent: Powerful, fresh, & woody-herbaceous

Blends Will With: Bergamont, Black Pepper, Cedarwood, Cinnamon, Citronella, Clary Sage, Eucalyptus, Frankincense, Geranium, Grapefruit Pink, Lavender, Lemon, Mandarin, Marjoram, Peppermint, Petitgrain, Pine, Tea Tree, and Thyme

Cautions: *Do not apply on or near the face of infants or children.*

Rosemary is stimulating, warming, and refreshing and can be used to help boost memory retention and staying alert. It has many skin care applications, including adding to a shampoo to aid in maintaining a healthy scalp and lustrous hair.

When diffused, Rosemary can also be helpful as a respiratory support oil. Rosemary is also beneficial in massage blends, increasing circulation and warmth to the skin and underlying muscles.

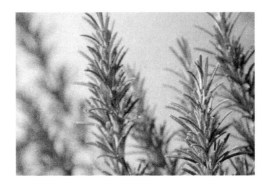

Rosemary

Sandalwood Essential Oil

Botanical Name: Santalum spicatum

Country of Origin: Australia

Extraction Method: Steam Distilled

Plant Part: Wood

Strength of Aroma: Medium

Aromatic Scent: A soft, sweet woody scent

Blends Well With: Bergamot, Cedarwood Virginian, Copaiba Balsam, Coriander Seed, Geranium, Lemon, Mandarin, Neroli, Palmarosa, Patchouli, Rose Absolute and Vetiver.

Sandalwood Australian is a precious oil that has been cherished for centuries by its users. This gentle oil is effective for skin care, relieving tension, and calming agitated emotions. Sandalwood components are perfect to help reduce oily skin and skin blemishes.

Its rich, woodsy scent is strong, but has a hint of sweetness that makes this oil a dream to the senses. When diffused or inhaled, it is a favorite for meditation to help relax the mind from the worries of everyday life.

Spearmint Essential Oil

Botanical Name: Mentha spicata

Country of Origin: Northwest USA, China, South America, Japan

Extraction Method: Steam Distilled

Plant Part: Leaves-1 kg oil yield from: 50–100 kg of the semi-dried herb

Strength of Aroma: Medium

Aromatic Scent: Sweet mint scent

Blends Well With: Bergamot, Dill Weed, Jasmine Absolute, Lavender, Vanilla C02

Spearmint is a wonderful child safe oil from the same family as peppermint. When diluted in a carrier oil and applied to the abdomen, it can help relieve a queasy stomach and bloating. When diffused, Spearmint is uplifting, reduces emotional agitation, improves concentration, and eases physical tension in the head and neck.

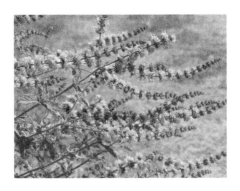

Spearmint

Spruce Black Essential Oil

Botanical Name: Picea mariana

Country of Origin: Canada

Extraction Method: Steam Distilled

Aromatic Scent: Fresh, Crisp, Woody and Earthy

Blends Well With: Bergamot, Cedarwood, Frankincense, Lavender, Lemon,

Spruce Black is an abundant evergreen tree that produces an essential oil loaded with therapeutic properties. Historically, Spruce Black has been used in ointments, salves, and lotions to help soothe muscular discomfort and to ease tight breathing associated with seasonal concerns and pollen threats.

With its fresh and uplifting aroma, it also helps lift away feelings of the winter doldrums by fighting off fatigue and energizing the senses.

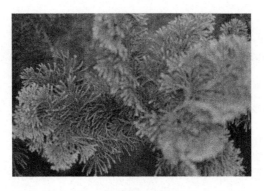

Spruce

Tangerine Essential Oil

Botanical Name: Citrus reticulata

Country of Origin: Brazil, Mexico

Extraction Method: Cold Pressed

Plant Part: Fruit Peel

Strength of Aroma: Medium

Aromatic Scent: Tangerine has a fresh, sweet citrus scent

Blends Well With: Bergamot, Clary Sage, Coriander Seed, Cypress, Geranium Grapefruit Pink, Lavender, Lemon, Lime, Neroli, Orange Sweet, Petitgrain, Rose Absolute and Vanilla CO2.

Tangerine is bright, refreshing, and rejuvenating. Its brightness can help clear the mind and reduce nervous tension. It is also a helpful support to the immune system. Additionally, Tangerine can help quell digestive issues such as a queasy stomach when added to a carrier oil and applied to the abdomen.

Tea Tree Essential Oil

Botanical Name: Melaleuca alternifolia

Country of Origin: Australia

Extraction Method: Steam distilled

Plant Part: Leaves/twigs-1 kg oil yield from: 60 kg of leaves and twigs

Strength of Aroma: Medium

Aromatic Scent: Fresh, medicinal, green wood scent

Blends Well With: Bergamot, Cypress, Grapefruit Pink, Juniper Berry, Lavender, Lemon, Marjoram Sweet, Pine Scots, Rose Absolute,

Tea Tree essential oil is one of the most popular essential oils, and for good reason. Native to Australia, it is commonly applied around the world for a multitude of uses.

It has a green, medicinal, woody aroma and is a wonderful addition to natural home-cleaning sprays and can clear and refresh musty areas. This oil is also fabulous for helping to clear teenage blemishes and other problem skin areas.

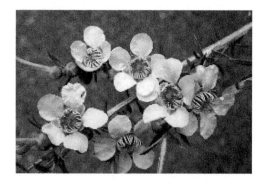

Tea Tree

Thyme Essential Oil

Botanical Name: Thymus Vulgaris

Country of Origin: France, Spain, United States

Extraction Method: Steam Distilled

Plant Part: Aerial Parts

Strength of aroma: Medium

Blends Well With: Grapefruit Pink, Lavender, Lemon, Marjoram Sweet, Oregano, Pine, Rosemary, and Vetiver

Thyme essential oils is known as one of the best oils for supporting the immune system. This powerful oil is also great for assisting the occasional digestive upset. It can also be used during seasonal illness to help clear the respiratory tract; just apply a couple of drops to a diffuser.

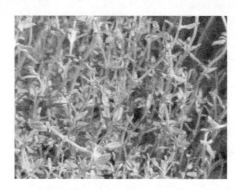

Thyme

Vanilla Oleoresin Essential Oil

Botanical Name: Vanilla planifolia

Country of Origin: Madagascar

Extraction Method: Solvent extraction

Plant Part: Seeds

Strength of Aroma: Medium

Aromatic Scent: A soft, sweet, rich and full scent

Blends Well With: Bergamot, Grapefruit Pink, Jasmine Absolute,

Lemon, Mandarin, Orange Sweet, Rose Absolute, Sandalwood, Tangerine, Vanilla CO2, Vetiver.

Vanilla Oleoresin is well known for its warm, inviting scent and is often used in sensual blends. When added to a carrier oil, it can help reduce nervous tension and agitation, and promote relaxation before sleep. Its rich, comforting, familiar aroma makes a wonderful addition to many DIY aromatherapy products.

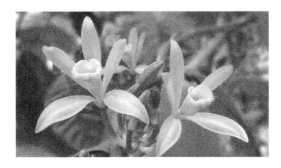

Vanilla

Vetiver Essential Oil

Botanical Name: Vetiveria zizanioides

Country of Origin: South India (native), Sri Lanka (native), West Java (native), Madagascar, Réunion, Haiti, China, Brazil.

Extraction Method: Steam distilled

Plant Part: Roots-1 kg oil yield from: 50 kg of roots

Strength of Aroma: Strong

Aromatic Scent: Powerful earthy, woody, smoky scent

Blends Well With: Bergamot, Clary Sage, Cypress, Frankincense, Helichrysum Italicum, Lavender, Lemon, Marjoram Sweet, Patchouli, Black Pepper, Rose Absolute, Sandalwood, Turmeric CO2.

Vetiver is a root oil that is abundant with therapeutic properties. This oil is known for its ability to promote relaxation and balance.

Vetiver can be used before bedtime to help calm the mind. It has an extraordinarily strong aroma that has an earthy, woodsy, smoky scent, but is pleasant to the senses.

Vetiver has been used in natural perfumery for years because of its unique aroma and only a small amount is needed to smell that amazing aroma. Its gentle and effective qualities will help skin blemishes as well as support a healthy immune system.

Ylang Ylang Essential Oil

Botanical Name: Cananga Odorata

Country of Origin: India (native), Philippines, Malaysia, Indonesia, and parts of Australia

Extraction Method: Steam distilled

Plant Part: Flowers- 2% yield from flowers

Aromatic Scent: fruity, flowery, and rich

Blends Well With: Bergamont, Geranium, Grapefruit, Lemon, Marjoram, Sandalwood, Vetiver

Ylang Ylang, known as the cananga tree is a tropical tree native to India. This beautiful, star shaped yellow flower is known for its potent aroma and is used in many commercial products for skin and hair, perfumes, massage oils, perfumes, and colognes.

This popular oil is also known to reduce depression, boost mood, alleviate anxiety, lower blood pressure, and decrease heart rate.

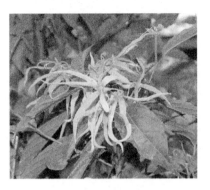

Ylang Ylang

The "Essential" Essential Oils

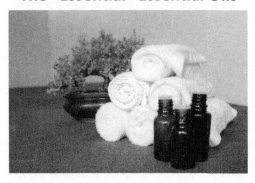

The following is a list of recommend essential oils that are great to have in your collection. Known for their numerous benefits, these are wonderful "go to" oils.

Cardamom *(Elettara Cardamomum)*   *Use For:*

- Bacteria
- Bad Breath
- Cavities
- Digestive Issues
- Energizing
- Fungii
- Pain and Inflammation

Chamomile Roman *(Anthemis Nobilis)*   *Use For:*

- Allergy Relief
- Calming
- Insomnia
- Pain
- PMS Symptoms
- Skin Disorders

Eucalyptus Radiata *(Eucalyptus Radiata)*   *Use For:*

- Bites and Stings
- Cuts

	• Cold and Flu
	• Energizing and Stimulating
	• Cleaning
Frankincense *(Boswellia Carterii)*	*Use For:*
	• Astringent
	• Cold/Flu Medicine
	• Natural Cleaner
	• Pain
	• Skin Disorders
	• Stomach Issues
	• Stress Reliever
Geranium *(Pelargonium Graveolens)*	*Use For:*
	• Abrasions/Cuts/Injuries
	• Depression and Stress
	• Infections
Lavender *(Lavandula Angustifolia)*	*Use For:*
	• Air Freshener
	• Antioxidant Protection
	• Beneficial for Skin
	• Headaches
	• Healing Cuts and Burns
	• Insomnia
	• Improving Mood
Lemon *(Citus Limon)*	*Use For:*
	• Bad Breath
	• Cleansing
	• Stomach Issues
	• Quenching Thirst
Peppermint *(Mentha Piperita)*	*Use For:*
	• Concentration

	<ul><li>Cooling</li><li>Halitosis (Bad Breath)</li><li>Headaches</li><li>Pain</li><li>Stomach Issues</li></ul>
Rosemary *(Rosmarinus Officinalis)*	*Use For:* <ul><li>Concentration</li><li>Hair Growth</li><li>Memory</li><li>Pain</li></ul>
Tea Tree *(Boswellia Carterii)*	*Use For:* <ul><li>Acne</li><li>Cleaning Products</li><li>Deodorant</li><li>Hair and Dandruff</li><li>Infections and Cuts</li><li>Mold</li><li>Skin Issues</li><li>Toenail Fungus and Ringworm</li></ul>
Thyme Linalol (Thymus Vulgaris Ct. Linalool)	*Use For:* <ul><li>Bacteria</li><li>Bronchitis and Cough</li><li>Fungii</li><li>High Blood Pressure</li><li>Sore Throat</li><li>Preventing Food Poisoning</li></ul>

Where to Buy Your Essential Oils

With so many essential oils on the market nowadays, it can be difficult to know what brand of essential oils to purchase and how to know if your oils are pure. Many essential oils sold online are mixed with other fillers. Pure essential oils should not be "oily" hence their name.

One test you can do to see if your essential oils are pure is to put a couple of drops on a piece of paper and hold up to the light. There should not be a "greasy" mark.

Another way to know if your oils are pure is to look at the label on the bottle. (See label below) The label should include the following:

- Common Name (i.e. lavender, peppermint)
- Latin Name (exact species or genus)
- Country of Origin
- Part of Plant Processed
- Type of Extraction (distillation or expression)
- How it was grown (traditional, wild-crafted, organic)

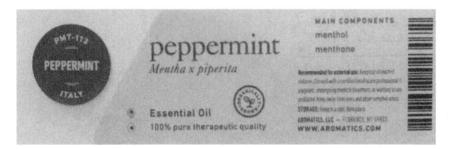

Any finally, look for companies that specialize in essential oils. Some examples of reputable companies are:

Aromatics International- **https://www.aromatics.com/**

Rocky Mountain Oils- https://www.rockymountainoils.com/

Plant Therapy Essential Oils- **https://www.planttherapy.com/**

Aura Cacia Essential Oils- **https://www.auracacia.com/**

Now Foods Essential Oils- **https://www.nowfoods.ca/essential-oils**

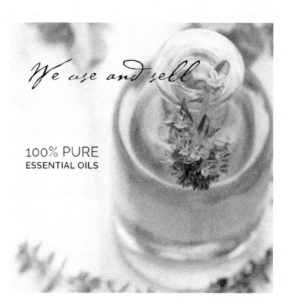

Essential Oil Dilution Chart

Dilution Guidelines for Essential Oils

*Values are approximate and have been rounded to whole drops. For essential oil blends, the numbers represent the total number of drops for all combined oils.

Please Note: All these dilutions may not be safe for all essential oils in all situations.

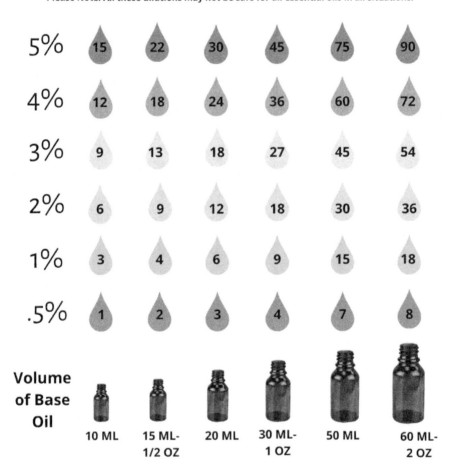

	10 ML	15 ML- 1/2 OZ	20 ML	30 ML- 1 OZ	50 ML	60 ML- 2 OZ
5%	15	22	30	45	75	90
4%	12	18	24	36	60	72
3%	9	13	18	27	45	54
2%	6	9	12	18	30	36
1%	3	4	6	9	15	18
.5%	1	2	3	4	7	8

Volume of Base Oil

Essential Oil Shelf Life

Listed below is a basic break down for the shelf life of your essential oils. Degradation comes about from three main ways: light, heat, and oxygen. For this reason, it is best to store your essential oils in the refrigerator or a dark cool place in dark glass bottles.

Carrier oils and carrier blends can be stored in PET plastic containers.

In general, shelf life is determined by the chemical composition of the essential oils, some of which oxidize or evaporate faster than others.

- The essential oils which have a lot of monoterpenes or oxides have the shortest shelf life, which is around about 1 -3 years.
- The Essential oils that contain ketones, monoterpenols, and/or esters usually have a shelf life of 3-5 years.
- The Essential oils that contain lots of sesquiterpenes and sesquiterpenes have a shelf life of 6-8 years or longer.

Common Essential Oils Shelf Life

- 1-3 years: Lemon, Frankincense, Tea Tree
- 3-5 years: Basil Sweet, Clary Sage, Geranium
- 6-8 years or longer: Cedarwood, Vetiver, Patchouli

If oils are not stored properly, their shelf life decreases significantly so be sure to store them in a dark cool place or keep them in the fridge.

If you have any expired oils or oils that are close to reaching the end of their shelf life, use them for cleaning! Add them to your cleaning blend sprays! There are some great cleaning spray recipes in the Cleaning Naturally section of this book!

CHAPTER 3: ESSENTIAL OIL BLENDING BASICS

"Health is the state about which medicine has nothing to say."
- W. H. Auden

Based on their aromas, essential oils can be categorized into different groups. Oils in the same category generally blend well together.

• Floral (i.e. Lavender, Rose, Jasmine)

• Woodsy (i.e. Pine, Cedar, Sandalwood)

• Earthy (i.e. Vetiver, Patchouli)

• Herbaceous (i.e. Rosemary, Basil)

• Minty (i.e. Peppermint, Spearmint)

• Medicinal/Camphorous (i.e. Eucalyptus, Tea Tree)

• Spicy (i.e. Clove, Cinnamon)

• Oriental (i.e. Ginger, Patchouli)

• Citrus (i.e. Orange, Bergamont, Lemon)

• *Florals blend well with spicy, citrusy, and woodsy oils.*

• *Woodsy oils generally blend well with all categories.*

• *Spicy and oriental oils blend well with florals, oriental and citrus oils.*

• *Minty oils blend well with citrus, woodsy, herbaceous, and earthy oils.*

Essential Oil Blends for Specific Emotions

The Top, Middle and Base Notes in Blending:

• Oils that evaporate the quickest, usually within 1-2 hours, are called **"top notes."** The top note is the first smell to arise from the blend. This note's fragrance is usually light, airy, and penetrating. Top notes stimulate and clear the mind, uplifting your energy.

• Oils that evaporate within 2-4 hours are considered **"middle notes."** The middle note also called the "heart note" gives the blend aromatic softness and can round off any sharp edges. This note provides balance both physically and energetically. Middle notes are soothing and harmonizing to the mind and the body.

• Oils that take the longest time to evaporate are referred to as **"base notes."** They function by reducing the evaporation of the top notes. Base notes often have an earthy aroma and add intensity to the blend. Unlike top notes, which penetrate quickly, the aroma of the base note rises slowly to your nose. Base note oils provide a warm, grounding quality to the blend. Most base note oils are derived from woods, resins, or roots.

Tip: When creating a new blend, start out with a total number of drops of either 6, 12, 18, or 24. 24 drops should be the most you start with as you don't want to waste your oils.

When blending, add one drop at a time, mix and smell. Allow the blend to unfold slowly. Doing this will inform you what oils you need to add and how much. You often need much less than you think.

Use caution with strong floral essential oils such as Geranium, Neroli, Rose Absolute, and Ylang Ylang. With these powerful oils, you only need to add 1-3 drops to a blend.

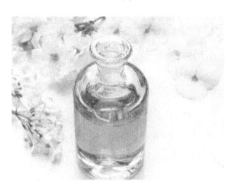

Calming/Soothing Essential Oils

Top Note	Middle Note	Base Note
Bergamont	Balsam Fir	Benzoin
Cajeput	Cardamom	Cedarwood
Clary Sage	Roman Chamomile	Frankincense
Coriander	Cypress	Ginger
Lemongrass	Fir Needle	Jasmine
Orange	Geranium	Myrrh
Petitgrain	Lavender	Patchouli
Spearmint	Marjoram	Rose
Tangerine	Melissa	Rosewood
Tea Tree	Myrtle	Sandalwood
	Neroli	Valerian
	Nutmeg	Vanilla
	Thyme	Vetiver
		Violet

		Ylang Ylang

Concentration/Memory

Top Note	Middle Note	Base Note
Basil	Rosemary	Frankincense
Peppermint		Ylang Ylang
Lemon		
Orange		

Anger

Top Note	Middle Note	Base Note
Bergamont	Roman Chamomile	Jasmine
Orange	Neroli	Patchouli
Petitgrain	Palmarosa	Rose
		Vetiver
		Ylang Ylang

Loneliness/Discontent/Grief/Helplessness

Top Note	Middle Note	Base Note
Bergamont	Chamomile	Benzoin
Grapefruit	Lavender	Frankincense
Lemon	Neroli	Helichrysum

Orange		Jasmine
Tangerine		Rose
Lime		Sandalwood

Stress/Anxiety

Top Note	Middle Note	Base Note
Bergamont	Roman Chamomile	Benzoin
Clary Sage	Geranium	Cedarwood
Orange	Juniper Berry	Frankincense
Coriander	Lavender	Jasmine
Grapefruit	Neroli	Patchouli
Mandarin	Pine	Rose
Petitgrain	Thyme	Sandalwood
		Valerian
		Ylang Ylang
		Helichrysum

Exhausted/Overwhelmed

Top Note	Middle Note	Base Note
Basil	Clary Sage	Ginger
Bergamont	Cinnamon	Frankincense
Coriander	Juniper Berry	Helichrysum

Eucalyptus	Palmarosa	Jasmine
Grapefruit	Peppermint	Sandalwood
Lemon	Rosemary	Ylang Ylang
Orange		
Tangerine		

Stimulating

Top Note	Middle Note	Base Note
Aniseed	Bay	Ginger
Basil	Black Pepper	Jasmin
Camphor	Cardamom	Myrrh
Citronella	Caraway Seed	Patchouli
Coriander	Cinnamon	Tarragon
Eucalyptus	Clove Bud	
Fennel	Dill	
Grapefruit	Geranium	
Lemon	Juniper Berry	
Lime	Lavender	
Mandarin	Marjoram	
Orange	Myrtle	
Oregano	Nutmeg	
Palmarosa	Pine	

Peppermint	Rosemary	
Rosemary Verbena	Thyme	
Sage		
Spearmint		

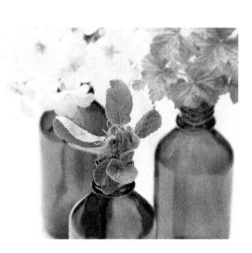

Additional Essential Oil Blends

Antifungal

Top Note	Middle Note	Base Note
Basil	Chamomile, German	Cedarwood
Bay Laurel	Cinnamon	Frankincense
Bergamont	Cypress	Helichrysum
Cajeput	Geranium	Myrrh
Citronella	Juniper Berry	Patchouli
Eucalyptus	Lavender	Rose
Grapefruit	Marjoram	Rosewood
Lemon	Melissa	Sandalwood
Lemongrass	Myrtle	Tarragon
Lime	Palmarosa	Vetiver
Orange	Pine	
Oregano	Rosemary	
Peppermint	Spruce	
Petitgrain	Thyme	
Tea Tree		

Anti-Bacterial

Top Note	Middle Note	Base Note
Basil	Black Pepper	Cedarwood
Bay Laurel	Cinnamon	Frankincense
Bergamont	Clove Bud	Ginger
Cageput	Chamomile	Helichrysum
Citronella	Cypress	Myrrh
Clary Sage	Geranium	Patchouli
Coriander	Juniper Berry	Rose
Eucalyptus	Lavender	Rosewood
Garlic	Marjoram	Sandalwood
Grapefruit	Melissa	Tarragon
Lemon	Myrtle	Valerian
Lemongrass	Neroli	Vetiver
Lemon Myrtle	Palmarosa	
Lime	Pine	
Mandarin	Rosemary	
Orange	Spruce	
Oregano	Thyme	
Peppermint		
Petitgrain		
Sage		

Tangerine		
Tea Tree		

Antiseptic

Top Note	Middle Note	Base Note
Aniseed	Bay	Balsam
Basil	Black Pepper	Benzoin
Bay Laurel	Caraway Seed	Cedarwood
Bergamont	Carrot Seed	Frankincense
Cajeput	Cinnamon	Ginger
Camphor	Clove Bud	Helichrysum
Citronella	Cypress	Jasmine
Clary Sage	Chamomile	Myrrh
Coriander	Geranium	Patchouli
Eucalyptus	Juniper Berry	Rose
Fennel	Lavender	Rosewood
Garlic	Marjoram	Sandalwood
Grapefruit	Melissa	Tarragon
Lemon	Myrtle	Vetiver
Lemongrass	Neroli	Ylang Ylang
Lime	Nutmeg	
Mandarin	Palmarosa	

Orange	Peppermint	
Oregano	Pine	
Peppermint	Rose Geranium	
Sage	Thyme	

Antiviral

Top Note	Middle Note	Base Note
Basil	Cinnamon	Cedarwood
Bergamont	Clove Bud	Frankincense
Cajeput	Cypress	Ginger
Coriander	Geranium	Helichrysum
Eucalyptus	Juniper Berry	Myrrh
Fennel	Lavender	Patchouli
Garlic	Marjoram	Rose
Grapefruit	Melissa	Rosewood
Lemon	Myrtle	Sandalwood
Lemongrass	Palmarosa	
Lime	Pine	
Mandarin	Rosemary	
Orange	Spruce	
Oregano	Thyme	
Peppermint		

Petitgrain		
Sage		
Tea Tree		

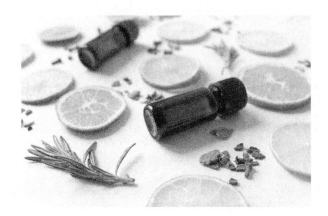

CHAPTER 5: CARRIER OIL PROPERTIES

"To keep the body in good health is a duty...otherwise we shall not be able to keep our mind strong and clear." -Buddha

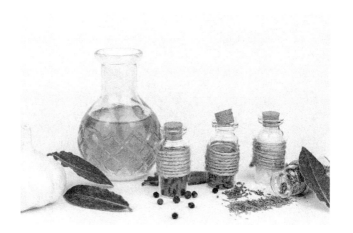

Benefits of Different Carrier Oils

Carrier Oils	Benefits
Nut Oils: Almond Hazelnut Macadamia Walnut	Anti-inflammatory Extremely soothing and emollient great for sensitive, dry, and inflamed skin Efficient in face mask treatments for acne-prone skin Maintaining skin elasticity and tightness Facilitates wound healing
Essential Fatty Acid Oils: Argan Babassu Calendula	Anti-inflammatory, Anti-bacterial, Anti-fungal Hydrating and soothing to dry, itchy, inflamed, and acne-prone skin Facilitate wound healing with reparative and astringent properties Balance hormones Balance essential fatty acid deficiency and skin's oil production

Fruit Oils:	Moisturizing without leaving a greasy residue due to the light texture
Apricot	
	Nourishing; suitable for sensitive skin
Avocado	
	Reduce the appearance of aging skin
Grape Seed	
	Cleansing and softening
Peach Kernel	
	Exhibits antioxidant properties
Olive	
Seed Oils:	Repair damage caused by dryness
Baobab	Rejuvenate complexion, especially in mature or prematurely aging skin
Black Currant	
	Reduce appearance of scarring
Borage	
	Soothe discomfort caused by burns
Broccoli	
Carrot	

Different Carrier Oils and Absorption Rates

Carrier Oil	Description	Absorption Rate
Avocado (CP, Refined) Black Currant Seed Carrot (CP, Macerated) Castor Flax Seed (CP) Oat Olive (CP, Extra Virgin) Pomegranate (CP, Refined) Sea Buckthorn (CO2) Shea Butter Sunflower (CP) Sweet Almond (CP, Virgin) Tamanu (CP, Madagascar) (CP- Cold Pressed)	These oils tend to feel waxy or gummy before warming up to the body temperature. They also tend to leave a slight oily residue on the skin.	SLOW
Argan Babassu Cocoa Butter Hemp Seed (CP, Unrefined)	These oils leave a silky feeling on the skin.	AVERAGE

Jojoba (CP) Raspberry Seed Sesame		
Apricot Kernel (CP) Broccoli Seed Camellia Seed (CP) Canola Fractionated Coconut Grape Seed Mango Butter Meadowfoam Prickly Pear	These oils are light and are quickly absorbed by the skin but leave a smooth, silky finish. Skin will feel moisturized but not greasy.	FAST
Hazelnut (CP) Rosehip (CP, Extra Virgin)	These oils are drying due to quick absorption into the skin and don't leave a greasy residue. High in polyunsaturated fat	VERY FAST

Shelf Life of Common Carrier Oils

Almond Oil (refined, expeller pressed) – 1 year	Jojoba Oil (cold pressed) – 5 years
Aloe Vera Oil – 6 months – 1 year	Macadamia Nut Oil (cold pressed) – 1 year
Apricot Kernel Oil (cold pressed) – 1 year	Moringa Seed Oil – 1+ years
Argan Oil (cold pressed/unrefined) – 2+ years	Neem Oil (cold pressed/unrefined) – 2 years
Avocado Oil (cold pressed/unrefined) – 1 year	Olive Oil (cold pressed/unrefined) – 2 years
Borage Oil – 6 months (may go rancid more quickly if not refrigerated)	Palm Oil (Red – unrefined) – 2 years
Brazil Nut Oil – 2 years	Papaya Seed Oil (cold pressed) – 1 year
Calendula Oil (infused) – 1 year	Passion Fruit Seed Oil (Maracuja Oil – cold pressed) – 1-2 years
Camellia Oil – 2 years	Peach Kernel Oil (cold pressed/unrefined) – 1 year
Carrot Seed Oil (cold pressed) – 1 year	Pecan Nut Oil (cold pressed/unrefined) – 1 year
Castor Oil (cold pressed) – 5 years	Pomegranate Seed Oil – 1 year
Chia Seed Oil (cold pressed) – 2 years	Poppy Seed Oil – 1 year
Coconut Oil (cold pressed/unrefined) – 2-4 years	Rose Hip Seed Oil – 6 months (refrigerated)

Cranberry Seed Oil – 2 years	Safflower Seed Oil (high linoleic) – 2 years
Emu Oil – 1 year (refrigerated)	Safflower Seed Oil (high oleic) – 2 years
Evening Primrose Oil (cold pressed) – 6 months – 1 year	Sesame Oil (cold pressed) – 1 year
Flax Seed Oil – 6 months (refrigerated)	Shea Oil – 1 year
Fractionated Coconut Oil – 5+ years	Soybean Oil (refined) – 1 year
Grapeseed Oil (cold pressed) – 1 year	Sunflower Seed Oil (cold pressed/unrefined) – 1 year
Hazelnut Oil (cold pressed) – 1 year	Tamanu Oil (cold pressed/unrefined) – 1 year
Hemp Seed Oil (cold pressed) – 1 year (refrigerated)	Walnut Oil (unrefined) – 2 years
Hypericum Oil (St John's Wort – infused) – 1 year	Wheat Germ Oil (unrefined) – 1 year

Many Uses of Coconut Oil

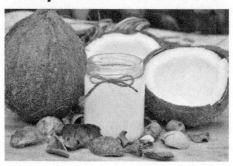

Wow! Did you know there were so many beneficial uses of coconut oil? This magnificent oil can benefit your body in so many ways. Check out the many uses below:

Cooking: Coconut oil is a great substitute for vegetable oil, olive oil, or butter.

Moisturizer: Put coconut oil on your body after showering or bathing for silky, smooth skin.

Hair Conditioner: Coconut oil helps repair damaged hair. Apply 1 tsp. of coconut oil to your hair. Leave in your hair approximately 15 minutes before shampooing it out.

Dandruff Treatment: Mix 1 tsp. coconut oil with 3 drops of tea tree essential oil. Massage into scalp and wait approximately 5 minutes before shampooing it out.

Bath Melts: Mix 1 cup coconut oil with 15–20 drops of your favorite essential oil(s). Freeze in a silicone mold. Drop one in your next bath!

Shaving Cream: Simply apply coconut oil over legs before shaving. It's not only a shaving cream but it also will act as an after-shave moisturizer as well.

Massage Oil: You can use coconut oil alone, but I personally think that it is better to combine it with another carrier oil (50/50)

Sugar Scrub: Mix coconut oil, brown sugar, and peppermint oil for a refreshing lip or skin scrub.

Acne: Apply a small amount of coconut oil after washing your face with soap and water. At first, your complexion may get worse as toxins are expelled from the skin but then it should improve after some time.

Chafe Protection: Use a little coconut oil to soothe chafing.

Surface Polisher: Use coconut oil to polish stainless steel, bronze, leather, furniture, wood, and artificial plants.

Wood Conditioner: Rub coconut oil on wooden utensils to help condition them. Add a few drops of lemon essential oil to help sanitize wood cutting boards and utensils.

Bruises and Minor Burns: Apply something cold (ice for bruises; cold, wet cloth for burns) for 10–15 minutes. Then gently apply a layer of coconut oil with lavender essential oil. Re-apply oil 4–8 times a day, or every couple of hours, until the pain is gone or until healed.

Indigestion: For acute cases of indigestion, take 2 Tbsp. of coconut oil internally. If needed, take 1 Tbsp. again 6 hours later.

Oil Pulling: Swish 1 tsp of coconut oil in your mouth for 5 minutes daily. Not only does this help keep your breath fresh, but it will also aid in keeping those pearly white teeth. It will also pull toxins out of your body.

Itchy Skin/Psoriasis/Eczema: Massage warm coconut oil into affected area. Do it every couple of days.

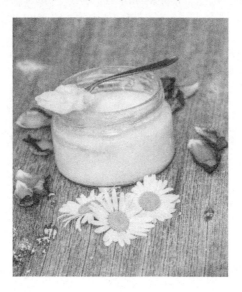

Conclusion

"Learning is the beginning of wealth. Learning is the beginning of health. Learning is the beginning of spirituality. Searching and learning is where the miracle process all begins." - Jim Rohn

Now that you have knowledge about aromatherapy, numerous essential oils, dilution, and blending we will move on to the second part of the book. This is the exciting part where you will learn how to make your own skin care products, pain relieving balms, and more! Enjoy!

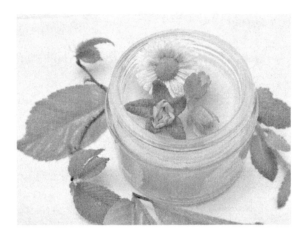

PART II: RECIPES USING ESSENTIAL OILS

"Health is the greatest gift, contentment the greatest wealth, faithfulness the best relationship." -Buddha

This is the fun part of the book where you will learn how to make your very own skin care products to use on yourself or others, balms and salves, foot, and body scrubs, and more! Below is a list of what will be covered:

- Diffuser Blends

- Aromatherapy Inhalers

- Air Freshener Sprays

- Aromatherapy Candles

- Roller Bottle Blends

- Body Scrubs & Foot Scrubs

- Bath Salts & Bath Bombs

- Foaming Body Wash

- Muscle Balms/Tiger Balms/Lip Balms

- Body Massage Lotions & Body Massage Oils

- Serum Blends for the Face

- Insect Repellents

Diffuser Blends

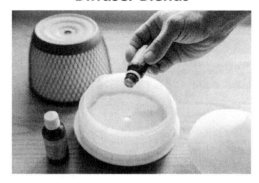

Note: To get the full therapeutic benefits, run your diffuser in 30-minute increments only. I recommend an ultra-sonic diffuser.

Refreshing Air Blends	Earthy Blends	Energy Boosting Blends
2 drops lemon 5 drops tea tree 4 drops clove	3 drops cedarwood 4 drops white fir 4 drops frankincense	3 drops rosemary 3 drops peppermint 4 drops lemon
5 drops lavender 3 drops lemon 2 drops rosemary	4 drops sandalwood 5 drops of pine	2 drops frankincense 3 drops cinnamon 4 drops bitter orange
3 drops lemon 2 drops tea tree 5 drops orange		2 drops peppermint 4 drops eucalyptus 4 drops grapefruit

3 drops peppermint 4 drops lemon 3 drops vetiver		
4 drops bergamot 3 drops grapefruit 3 drops lemon		

Citrusy/Zesty Blends	Elevating/Uplifting Blends	Immune Boosting Blends
2 drops lemon 2 drops bergamont 3 drops orange 3 drops grapefruit	2 drops lavender 4 drops geranium 4 drops bergamont	2 drops cinnamon 2 drops lemon 2 drops rosemary 4 drops eucalyptus
2 drops lime 2 drops grapefruit 3 drops lemon	2 drops spearmint 2 drops lemon 3 drops grapefruit	2 drops cinnamon bark 4 drops ginger 4 drops

3 drops sweet orange	3 drops lavender	frankincense
3 drops clove 3 drops cinnamon bark 4 drops sweet orange 2 drops lime 4 drops patchouli 4 drops sweet orange	2 drops frankincense 2 drops grapefruit 4 drops bitter orange	3 drops geranium 4 drops lavender 4 drops rosemary
		2 drops rosemary 2 drops clove 4 drops eucalyptus
		3 drops oregano 3 drops grapefruit 4 drops lemon

Headache Relief Blends	Focus/Concentration Blends	Stress Relief Blends
4 drops lavender 6 drops	2 drops rosemary 4 drops peppermint	2 drops ylang ylang

peppermint	4 drops basil	4 drops clary sage 4 drops lavender
2 drops eucalyptus 2 drops myrrh 6 drops peppermint	3 drops frankincense 3 drops rosemary 3 drops basil	4 drops frankincense 6 drops bergamont
3 drops lavender 3 drops tea tree 4 drops peppermint	2 drops lavender 3 drops basil 5 drops peppermint	2 drops geranium 3 drops roman chamomile 3 drops lavender
3 drops lavender 3 drops peppermint 4 drops ginger	3 drops peppermint 3 drops lemon 4 drops grapefruit	2 drops ylang ylang 2 drops chamomile 6 drops lavender

Cold & Flu Relief Blends	Insomnia Relief Blends
2 drops peppermint	2 drops ylang ylang
4 drops eucalyptus	4 drops bergamont
5 drops frankincense	4 drops patchouli

2 drops rosemary 2 drops eucalyptus 4 drops lemon 2 drops peppermint	4 drops sandalwood 6 drops lavender 3 drops chamomile
2 drops peppermint 3 drops lemon 4 drops lavender	3 drops vetiver 3 drops chamomile 4 drops lavender
2 drops peppermint 3 drops scots pine 3 drops lemon 3 drops spike lavender	2 drops chamomile 4 drops juniper 4 drops lavender
3 drops rosemary 3 drops juniper 4 drops frankincense	4 drops cedarwood 6 drops lavender

Aromatherapy Inhalers

Aromatherapy inhalers are great for a quick "pick me up", pesky allergies, or even fighting a cold or the flu. You can throw one in your purse or put in your pocket for easy access.

You can find the plastic inhalers and cotton inserts at Amazon or if you would like a fancy one, those are available as well. Below is a list of blends you can add to your inhalers. Just add the drops to the cotton insert and place into inhaler.

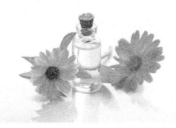

Uplifting Blends	Calming Blends	Allergy Relief Blends
10 drops geranium 8 drops bergamont	15 drops lavender 10 drops chamomile	10 drops eucalyptus radiata 10 drops rosemary ct. cineole 8 drops bay laurel
10 drops spearmint 8 drops lemon		10 drops tea tree 10 drops lemon 10 drops rosemary ct. cineole

Air Freshener Sprays

Purify your air or make your room smell delightful with a homemade room spritzer! Use distilled water and add approximately 40 drops of essential oils in a glass spray bottle. You can use more or less oil depending upon your preference of scent. Use 25% grain alcohol (Everclear) to the mixture to reduce microbial growth. The recipes below are for a 16 oz (500 ml) spray bottle:

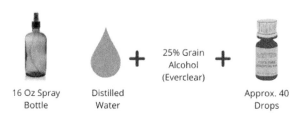

| 16 Oz Spray Bottle | Distilled Water | 25% Grain Alcohol (Everclear) | Approx. 40 Drops |

Herbal Delight	Fresh Forest	Beautiful Day	Saturday Afternoon	Cozy Day
20 drops lemon	10 drops pine	10 drops orange	15 drops lavender	20 drops wintergreen
5 drops rosemary	10 drops cedarwood	10 drops cedarwood	15 drops lime	10 drops lemongrass
5 drops thyme	10 drops lavender	10 drops lavender	5 drops spearmint	10 drops juniper berry
5 drops spearmint	10 drops spearmint	5 drops spearmint		
		5 drops frankincense		

Rejuvenating	Citrus Mint	Warming Spices	Holiday Harmony	Citrus Sensation
15 drops spearmint	20 drops lemon	15 drops orange	15 drops lavender	10 drops grapefruit
15 drops tangerine	5 drops basil	10 drops ginger	15 drops cedarwood	10 drops orange
10 drops bergamont	5 drops spearmint	10 drops ylang ylang	10 drops spruce	5 drops lemon
				5 drops bergamont

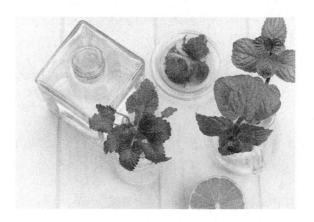

Aromatherapy Candles

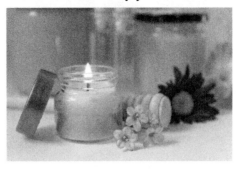

Aromatherapy candles are so easy and fun to make! Recycle your used jars and make a beautiful aromatherapy candle! They also make great gifts and who doesn't love a candle? The recipes below will be for an 8oz jar or tin.

If you decide you would like to make more than one candle at a time, I recommend purchasing a candle making pitcher which holds more wax. I normally purchase the wax, candle tins and wicks from Amazon due to their large selection but Bulk Apothecary also has a great selection of supplies.

Beeswax Aromatherapy Candle

- 8 oz jar or candle tin

- Beeswax Pellets

- Medium candle wick

- 6 ml of your preference of essential oil or a blend

Fill 8 oz jar or tin **1 ½ times** with beeswax pellets and pour into glass measuring cup. (Tip: For easier clean up, pour a little jojoba oil on a paper towel and wipe the inside of the glass measuring cup.)

Place measuring cup with pellets into pot of water filled ¼ of the way on medium low setting. (not boiling)

While wax is melting, place the wick in the center of the jar or tin and cut part of the wick if it's too long. **Tip:** You can use chopsticks to keep the wick from moving when you pour the wax or adhesive stickers to hold the wick in place.

Once wax is melted completely, stir in 6 ml of essential oils of your preference. You can use more or less depending upon your preference of scent. Pour into jar or tin. Set aside for a couple of hours and "voila" you have a beautiful candle ready for use!

Soy Aromatherapy Candle

- 8 oz jar or candle tin

- Medium candle wick

- 160 grams of soy wax (would recommend using a food scale if you have one)

- 6 ml of essential oil or your favorite oil or blend

Melt wax in a double boiler on medium low setting. (Pyrex measuring cup or pitcher in pot of water filled ¼ of the way)

While wax is melting, place the wick in the center of the jar or tin and cut part of wick if it's too long. You can use chopsticks to keep the wick from moving when your pour the wax, use adhesive stickers to hold the wick in place, or purchase wick holders.

Once wax is completely melted, stir in 6 ml of essential oils of your preference. You can use more or less depending upon preference of scent. Pour into jar or tin. Soy wax takes longer than beeswax to solidify so set aside for 24 hrs. before use.

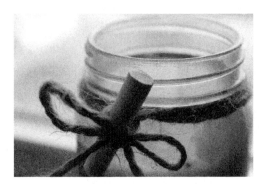

Roller Bottle Blends

Roller bottles are great to use for relief on specific areas of the body! The blends listed below are for a 10 ml glass roller bottle.

Add the essential oil and fill the rest of the bottle with a carrier oil of your choice and pop the roller cap on. Roll on your wrists or neck. (**Tip:** You may want to use a funnel to pour the carrier oil into the bottle.) Shake gently and use!

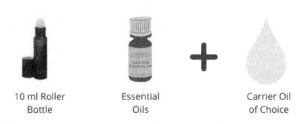

| 10 ml Roller Bottle | Essential Oils | Carrier Oil of Choice |

Muscle Aches	Stress Relief	Sleep Aid	Calm Your Mind	Chill Out
3 drops peppermint	4 drops peppermint	5 drops lavender	5 drops bergamot	4 drops lavender
3 drops wintergreen	2 drops frankincense	2 drops clary sage	5 drops frankincense	3 drops clary sage
2 drops lemongrass	2 drops lavender			2 drops ylang ylang
2 drops juniper	2 drops chamomile			1 drop marjoram

Itchy Bug Bites	Energy Booster	Focus & Concentration	Positivity	Acne Helper
3 drops lavender	3 drops orange	5 drops orange	3 drops grapefruit	4 drops lavender
3 drops peppermint	3 drops frankincense	5 drops peppermint	3 drops orange	4 drops melaleuca
2 drops frankincense	3 drops cinnamon		2 drops lemon	2 drops lemongrass
2 drops melaleuca			1 drop bergamont	
2 drops lemon				

Colds & Flu	Immune Booster	Upset Stomach	Headache Relief
4 drops peppermint	2 drops oregano	3 drops ginger	4 drops peppermint
2 drops eucalyptus	2 drops lemon	2 drops peppermint	4 drops lavender
2 drops lemon	2 drops frankincense	2 drops fennel	3 drops chamomile
2 drops rosemary	2 drops cinnamon	1 drop coriander	
	2 drops melaleuca	1 drop lemon	

Body Scrubs & Foot Scrubs

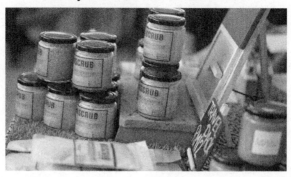

Pamper yourself with DIY Body and Foot scrubs! Scrubs will make your skin and feet feel silky soft plus they are great for exfoliating the skin. And they are so easy to make!

There are three main types of scrubs: **sugar, salt, and oatmeal**. Sugar is generally best for dry skin and salt is usually best for oily skin. Scoop a small amount into your hands and massage lightly to desired areas. Remove excess scrub with a warm, wet towel or shower afterwards and feel how soft and luxurious your skin feels!

Brown Sugar Body Scrub

- 1/2 cup brown sugar

- 2 Tbs jojoba oil

- 4 drops sandalwood essential oil

- 8 drops lavender essential oil

Mix and use.

Lemongrass Sugar Scrub

- 1 cup granulated sugar or brown sugar

- 1/3 cup jojoba oil

- 15 drops lemongrass essential oil

Combine and use.

Minty Salt Scrub

- 2 cups sea salt

- ¾ cup carrier oil of choice

- 10 drops peppermint essential oil

- 10 drops spearmint essential oil

- 10 drops lemon essential oil

Combine and use.

Chamomile Oatmeal Scrub

- ¾ cup granulated sugar

- ¼ cup ground raw oats

- ¼ cup coconut oil or carrier oil of choice

- 6 drops chamomile essential oil

- 4 drops geranium

Combine and use.

Revitalizing Foot Scrub

- 1 cup sea salt, Epsom salt, or brown sugar

- 1 tbsp coconut oil or carrier oil of choice

- 5 drops peppermint essential oil

- 5 drops tea tree essential oil

- 5 drops lavender essential oil

Mix and use (can store excess in airtight jar)

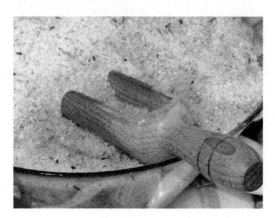

Bath Salts/Bath Bombs

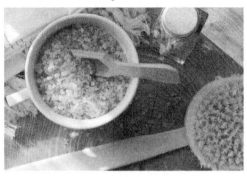

Looking to relax and unwind after a long day? There is nothing like an Epsom salt bath soak to escape and rejuvenate your body and ease those achy muscles!

Relax and Rejuvenate Epsom Salt Bath

- 2 cups of Epsom salt or Himalayan sea salt

- ½ cup of baking soda

- 2 tbsp of coconut oil or carrier oil of your choice

- 30 drops of lavender essential oil

- 10 drops of peppermint

Mix and add ¼ cup to ½ cup to bath water

Bath Bombs

- 1 cup baking soda

- ½ cup citric acid

- 1 cup of Epsom salt or sea salt

- 2 tbsp of coconut oil or carrier oil of choice

- 30 to 40 drops of essential oils of choice

- Spray bottle with water or witch hazel

Molds for bath bombs- You can use ice treys, greased muffin tins or if you prefer round molds, you can purchase round metal molds which are great! If you would like colored bath bombs you can use a small amount of food coloring.

Mix all the dry ingredients in a large bowl. Add the essential oils and carrier oil and mix. Spray the mixture with water or witch hazel until you get a "wet sand" consistency. Mixture should not crumble in your hands. (Use gloves if you have sensitive skin.)

Press the mixture into the molds and let sit for 24 to 48 hours to harden. Store in an airtight container.

If you are using the round tin molds, fill each half of the mold with mixture and then press the two halves together. Wipe off excess mixture on the outside and gently pull apart and place round bomb in hand and place on wax paper or aluminum foil to harden for 24hrs. (**Tip:** If the mixture falls apart when you take the bomb out of the mold, it's not wet enough. Place back into the bowl and spritz with more witch hazel or water.)

Foaming Body Wash

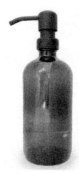 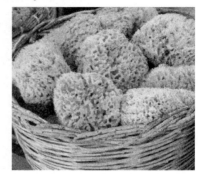

Save money and make your own foaming body wash! Plus, you can customize with your favorite essential oil blend!

You will just need a pump bottle to put your body wash in. Pump a few squirts onto a wet sponge and lather.

- 2/3 cup castile soap

- ¼ cup aloe gel

- 2 tbsp sweet almond oil or jojoba oil

- 1 tsp Vitamin E oil

- 50 – 60 drops of essential oils or blend of choice

Mix and pour into pump bottle

Muscle Balms/Tiger Balms/Lip Balms

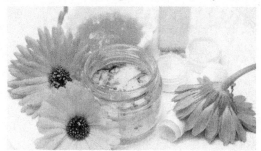

Achy Muscle Relief Balm

- ½ cup Coconut Oil

- ¼ cup Beeswax (grated or pellets)

- 2 tsp Turmeric Powder

- 2 tsp Cayenne Powder

- 8 drops Lavender essential oil

- 10 drops Peppermint essential oil

- 1 glass jar or container with lid

Melt the coconut oil and beeswax in a double boiler on medium low setting. (Glass Pyrex measuring cup in pot of water filled ¼ of the way) Add the turmeric and cayenne pepper and stir. Add the essential oils and stir. Pour into jar or tin.

Herbal Relief Salve

- 1 tbsp Beeswax (grated or pellets)

- 4 tbsp Coconut Oil

- 10 drops Peppermint essential oil

- 10 drops Eucalyptus essential oil

- 5 drops of Clove essential oil

Melt beeswax and coconut oil in double boiler on medium low setting. (Glass Pyrex measuring cup in pot of water filled ¼ of the way) Add the essential oils and stir. Pour into glass jar or container.

Tiger Balm

- 1 ¼ cup of Beeswax (shredded or pellets)

- ¼ cup Olive oil

- 5 drops Clove essential oil

- 5 drops Cinnamon essential oil

- 8 drops Eucalyptus essential oil

- 10 drops Peppermint essential oil

- 10 drops Camphor essential oil

Melt beeswax in double boiler on medium low setting. (Glass Pyrex measuring cup in pot of water filled ¼ of the way) and add olive oil and essential oils. Mix and pour into glass jar or container.

Athlete's Foot Salve

- ¼ cup Beeswax

- ¼ cup Extra Virgin Olive oil

- ¼ cup Almond oil

- ½ cup Shea Butter

- 40 drops Lavender essential oil

- 40 drops Tea Tree essential oil

- 1 glass jar

Melt the beeswax with the other oils in a double boiler on medium low setting. (Glass Pyrex measuring cup in pot of water filled ¼ of the way) Let cool slightly and add the essential oils. Pour into glass jar and use when needed.

Lemon Lip Balm

- 7 or 8 Lip balm containers

- 1 tbsp Beeswax (shredded or pellets)

- 1 tbsp Shea Butter or Cocoa butter

- 1 tbsp Coconut Oil

- 15-20 drops of Lemon essential oil or your preference

This recipe is for about 7 or 8 lip balms. I would recommend getting a trey to hold your lip balm containers as it's much easier to pour the mixture into the containers without them tipping over. You can purchase one from Amazon.

If you would like to make more lip balms, you can double the recipe. You can also use tins or small jars for your lip balm. The recipe may vary slightly depending on the size of the containers you are planning to use.

Melt Beeswax and Coconut oil first in a double boiler on medium low setting (Glass Pyrex measuring cup in pot of water filled ¼ of the way) and then add Shea Butter. Once melted, add the essential oil. Pour into lip balm containers.

Tip: The mixture hardens quickly so if you find your mixture is starting to solidify before you pour into all your containers, you can place back into the pot of water.

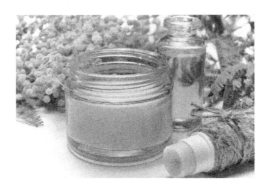

Body Massage Lotions & Body Massage Oils

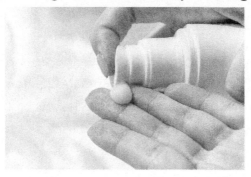

Relax Your Mind Lotion

• 6 drops Chamomile Roman essential oil

• 2 drops Neroli essential oil

• 2 drops Ylang Ylang essential oil

• 2 fl. oz. unscented lotion

• 2 oz. PET bottle with pop up cap or amber glass bottle

1% dilution- Safe for children 5 or older. Blend the essential in the lotion with a glass stir rod or metal spoon. Apply to your neck, throat, and chest. The ingredient with the shortest shelf life becomes the shelf life of the entire blend.

Muscle Spasm Relief Lotion

• 6 drops Petitgrain essential oil

• 3 drops Chamomile Roman essential oil

• 1 drop Ylang Ylang essential oil

• 1 drop Bergamont essential oil

- 1 fl. oz. unscented lotion

- 1 oz. glass jar

2% dilution- For children between the ages of 5 and 10, 2 drops of Petitgrain, 1 drop of Roman Chamomile, 1 drop of bergamont, and 1 drop of ylang ylang is recommended. Blend the essential oils with the lotion and use as needed for muscle cramps.

Calm and Balance Lotion

- 5 drops Lavender essential oil

- 4 drops Chamomile Roman essential oil

- 2 drops Vetiver essential oil

- 1 fl. oz. unscented lotion

- 1 oz. glass jar

2% dilution- For children between the ages of 5 and 10, 3 drops of lavender, 1 drop of vetiver, and 2 drops of roman chamomile is recommended. Blend all ingredients and apply to the wrists, hands, and neck.

Stress Relief Lotion

- 10 drops Lavender essential oil

- 8 drops Sandalwood essential oil

- 7 drops Chamomile Roman essential oil

- 2 fl. oz. of unscented lotion

- 2 oz. glass jar

2% dilution- For children between the ages of 5 and 10, use 5 drops of lavender, 4 drops sandalwood, and 3 drops of roman chamomile. Blend all ingredients and use as needed to relieve stress and emotional tension.

Menstrual Cramp Relief Lotion

- 6 drops Chamomile Roman essential oil

- 3 drops Bergamont essential oil

- 3 drops Lavender essential oil

- 3 drops Ylang Ylang essential oil

- 1 drop Rose Absolute essential oil

- 1 fl. oz. unscented lotion

- 1 oz. glass jar

3% dilution- Safe for kids 10 and up. Use precaution when going into the sun with Bergamont. Blend all the ingredients and massage into the cramp area several times a day.

Congestion Relief Lotion

- 9 drops Pine Scots essential oil

- 4 drops Mandarin essential oil

- 3 drops Eucalyptus Radiata essential oil

- 2 drops Cypress essential oil

- 1 fl. oz. unscented lotion

- 1 oz. glass jar

3% dilution- Safe for kids 10 and up. Asthmatics are recommended to gently smell cap prior to use to avoid any reaction. Blend all ingredients and massage into chest, neck, and upper back as needed for relief.

Immune Support Lotion

- 10 drops Cypress essential oil

- 10 drops Douglas Fir essential oil

- 5 drops Lemon essential oil

- 3 drops Tea Tree essential oil

- 2 fl. oz unscented lotion

- 2 oz. glass jar

2.5% dilution- Safe for kids 10 and up. Use cautions if asthmatic. Blend all ingredients and apply to neck, back, chest, and feet every couple of hours during initial signs of illness.

Muscle Tension Relief Oil

- 4 drops Rosemary essential oil

- 2 drops Frankincense essential oil

- 2 drops Black Pepper essential oil

- 1 drop Lemon essential oil

- 1 drop Bergamont essential oil

- 1 drop Juniper Berry essential oil

- 1 fl. oz. Jojoba Oil

- 1 oz glass bottle with dropper cap

2% dilution- Safe for kids 10 and up. Use caution if epileptic, pregnant, nursing, or going out into the sun. Blend all ingredients, place cap on bottle and shake gently. Apply to sore areas.

Relaxation and Rest Oil

- 8 drops Mandarin essential oil

- 6 drops Lavender essential oil

- 5 drops Chamomile Roman essential oil

- 1 fl. oz Jojoba Oil

- 1 oz. glass bottle with dropper cap

3% dilution- For children between the ages of 5 and 10, use 3 drops of mandarin, 2 drops of lavender, in 1 oz of carrier oil.

Massage gently into temples, chest, and upper back.

Skin Nourishing Oil

- 5 drops Orange Sweet essential oil

- 3 drops Geranium essential oil

- 2 drops Rose Absolute essential oil

- 1 drop Ylang Ylang essential oil

- 1 oz. Coconut Oil

- 1 oz. glass jar

2% dilution- Safe for children 10 and up. Blend all ingredients in glass jar and stir.

Moisturizing Hand Oil

- 6 drops Frankincense essential oil

- 6 drops Lavender essential oil

- 1 fl. oz. Sweet Almond Oil

- 1 oz. PET bottle with pop up cap

2% dilution- Safe for children 10 and up. Blend all ingredients in bottle and gently shake. Use as needed for dry hands.

Headache Relief Oil

- 5 drops Frankincense essential oil

- 4 drops Rosewood essential oil

- 3 drops Peppermint essential oil

- 2 drops Lemongrass essential oil

- 1 fl. oz Jojoba Oil

- 1 oz. glass bottle

2% dilution- Safe for children over 10. Blend all ingredients in bottle and gently shake. Apply to the back of your neck for the first few hours.

Immune Support Oil

- 9 drops Rosewood essential oil

- 4 drops Sandalwood essential oil

- 2 drops Lavender essential oil

- 1 fl. oz. Jojoba Oil

- 1 oz. glass bottle

3% dilution- Safe for children 10 and up. Blend all ingredients and shake gently. Apply to neck, chest and upper back as needed.

Soothing Joint Oil

- 5 drops Frankincense essential oil

- 3 drops Patchouli essential oil

- 2 drops Black Pepper essential oil

- 2 drops Lime essential oil

- 1 fl. oz. Arnica Oil

- 1 oz. glass bottle

2% dilution- Safe for kids 10 and up. Please use precautions if pregnant or nursing and avoid use on broken skin. Blend all ingredients and shake gently. Apply to painful joints as needed.

Serum Blends for the Face

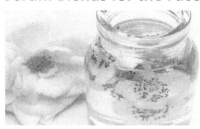

Best Carrier Oils for Your Skin Type

Normal	Dry	Oily	Sensitive	Mature	Acne Prone
Apricot Kernel	Avocado	Jojoba	Sunflower	Apricot Kernel	Argan
Jojoba	Sweet Almond	Argan	Jojoba	Avocado	Evening Primrose
Grapeseed	Rose Hip Seed	Grapeseed	Sweet Almond	Rose Hip Seed	Grapeseed
Sunflower	Apricot Kernel		Apricot Kernel	Jojoba	Jojoba
Sweet Almond	Sunflower		Rose Hip Seed	Sweet Almond	Sesame
			Avocado	Sunflower	
			Argan	Tamanu	
			Grapeseed		
			Evening Primrose		

Best Essential Oils for Skin Type

Normal	Dry	Oily	Mature	Non-Cystic Acne
Geranium	Clary Sage	Frankincense	Rose	Geranium
Frankincense	Cedarwood	Geranium	Frankincense	Cedarwood
Lavender	Geranium	Lavender	Myrrh	Lavender
	Myrrh	Patchouli	Helichrysum	Patchouli
	Rose	Tea Tree	Sandalwood	Tea Tree
	Jasmine	Ylang Ylang	Geranium	Rose
	Patchouli	Clary Sage	Lavender	Roman Chamomile
	Frankincense	Roman Chamomile	Patchouli	Lemongrass
	Roman Chamomile	Cypress	Cypress	Rosemary
	Ylang Ylang	Peppermint	Jasmine	
		Rosemary	Rosemary	
		Sandalwood		

Serum Blend Recipes

Please Note: In the following recipes, you can use any carrier oil or essential oil that suits your skin type, however, do not use more than 20 drops of essential oil. If you have sensitive skin, you should be more conservative with your essential oils and use 10 drops which would give you a 0.5% dilution.

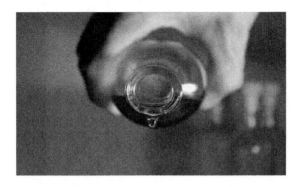

Face Serum for Normal Skin:

- 2 oz. (60 mls) bottle

- 2 oz. Apricot Kernel oil

- 8 drops Lavender essential oil

- 8 drops Geranium essential oil

- 4 drops Frankincense essential oil

Put lid on bottle and gently roll the bottle in the palm of your hand for about 30 seconds to mix the essential oils in with carrier oil. **To use:** Apply a drop of serum to forehead, each cheek, and chin. gently massage onto face using small, soft upward strokes.

Face Serum for Dry Skin:

- 2 oz. (60 mls) bottle

- 2 oz. Avocado oil

- 5 drops Rose essential oil

- 5 drops Jasmine essential oil

- 5 drops Frankincense essential oil

- 5 drops Geranium essential oil

Put lid on bottle and gently roll the bottle in the palm of your hand for about 30 seconds to mix the essential oils in with carrier oil. **To use:** Apply a drop of serum to forehead, each cheek, and chin. gently massage onto face using small, soft upward strokes.

Face Serum for Acne:

- 2 oz. (60 mls) bottle

- 2 oz. Jojoba Oil

- 5 drops Tea Tree essential oil

- 5 drops Lemongrass essential oil

- 10 drops Lavender essential oil

Put lid on bottle and gently roll the bottle in the palm of your hand for about 30 seconds to mix the essential oils in with carrier oil. **To use:** Apply a drop of serum to forehead, each cheek, and chin. gently massage onto face using small, soft upward strokes.

Face Serum for Sensitive Skin:

- 2 oz. (60 mls) bottle

- 1 oz. Jojoba

- 1 oz. Sweet Almond oil

- 5 drops Helichrysum essential oil

- 5 drops Sandalwood essential oil

- 5 drops Frankincense essential oil

- 5 drops Lavender essential oil

Put lid on bottle and gently roll the bottle in the palm of your hand for about 30 seconds to mix the essential oils in with carrier oil. **To use:** Apply a drop of serum to forehead, each cheek, and chin. gently massage onto face using small, soft upward strokes.

Face Serum for Oily Skin:

- 2 oz. (60 mls) bottle

- 1 oz. Jojoba Oil

- 1 oz. Argan oil

- 10 drops Cypress essential oil

- 5 drops Peppermint essential oil

- 5 drops Rosemary essential oil

Put lid on bottle and gently roll the bottle in the palm of your hand for about 30 seconds to mix the essential oils in with carrier oil. **To use:** Apply a drop of serum to forehead, each cheek, and chin. gently massage onto face using small, soft upward strokes.

Face Serum for Mature Skin:

- 2 oz. (60 mls) bottle

- 2 oz. Apricot Kernel oil

- 5 drops Rose essential oil

- 5 drops Helichrysum essential oil

- 5 drops Frankincense essential oil

- 5 drops Geranium essential oil

Put lid on bottle and gently roll the bottle in the palm of your hand for about 30 seconds to mix the essential oils in with carrier oil. **To use:** Apply a drop of serum to forehead, each cheek, and chin. gently massage onto face using small, soft upward strokes.

Face Serum for Combination Skin:

- 2 oz. (60 mls) bottle

- 1 oz. Jojoba oil

- 1 oz. Rose hip seed oil

- 5 drops Frankincense essential oil

- 5 drops Geranium essential oil

- 5 drops Lavender essential oil

- 5 drops Sandalwood essential oil

Put lid on bottle and gently roll the bottle in the palm of your hand for about 30 seconds to mix the essential oils in with carrier oil. **To use:** Apply a drop of serum to forehead, each cheek, and chin. gently massage onto face using small, soft upward strokes.

Insect Repellents

Make your own insect repellent free of harmful chemicals and keep those pesky bugs away! You can also add essential oils to a diffuser to keep those insects away!

Diffuser Insect Repellent

- 3 drops clove essential oil

- 3 drops cinnamon bark essential oil

- 4 drops lemongrass essential oil

Adult Insect Repellent

- 3% citronella essential oil

- 3% peppermint essential oil

- 4% turmeric essential oil

- 90% coconut oil

Child's Insect Repellent

- 3% citronella essential oil

- 3% ginger essential oil

- 4% turmeric essential oil

- 90% coconut oil

Conclusion

"Health is the soul that animates all the enjoyments of life, which fade and are tasteless without it." -Lucius Annaeus Seneca

I hope you enjoyed learning all the wonderful ways you can use essential oils and incorporate these beautiful oils into your daily living! In the next part you will learn how you can clean naturally with some awesome recipes!

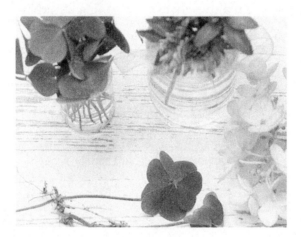

PART III: CLEANING NATURALLY

"What is called genius is the abundance of life and health." -Henry David Thoreau

Why spend a lot of money on cleaners full of harmful chemicals when you can use many products that you probably have under your sink or in your pantry? In this part of the book you will be learning some great alternatives for cleaning naturally!

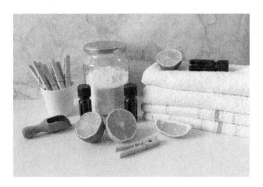

- White Vinegar Uses & Recipes

- Hydrogen Peroxide Uses

- Baking Soda Uses & Recipes

- Foaming Hand Cleanser

- Toilet Bowl Bombs

White Vinegar Uses & Recipes

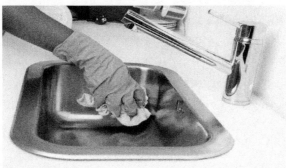

Who knew there were so many wonderful uses of white vinegar? This well-known addition to salad dressing has so many other beneficial uses!

Vinegar is great for cutting grease, disinfecting, and deodorizing! However, if you have natural stone countertops or flooring such as granite or marble, vinegar is not recommended. It also should not be used on cast iron or aluminum.

Note: Never mix vinegar with hydrogen peroxide! You can use them on the same surface separately while cleaning, but do not mix them in the same container. You will create a peracetic acid which is potentially irritating and corrosive.

For cleaning and disinfecting the kitchen sink, refrigerator, stove, microwave, bathroom sink, faucet handles etc., here is a great recipe you can make:

Cleaning and Disinfecting Spray

- Spray bottle

- 1 cup distilled water

- 1 cup vinegar

- 10 drops lemon essential oil

Treat Insect Bites and Stings

Dab white vinegar on mosquito bites and insect stings to relieve the pain of the sting and the itching. Vinegar will disinfect the area and facilitate healing.

Pet Urine on Carpet

Spray with 50/50 water and vinegar solution and blot with rag or paper towel. You can also sprinkle some baking soda to remove odor if necessary and vacuum afterwards.

Weed Killer

- 1-gallon white vinegar

- 1 Tbsp Epsom salts

- 2 Tbsp dish soap

- Spray onto weeds to kill them and pour into concrete cracks to stop them from growing back so quickly.

Remove Antiperspirant Stains

Apply white vinegar on a microfiber cloth and rub the stain.

Sanitize the Bathroom

A simple way to sanitize your bathroom is to spray everything with vinegar and the wipe it down with a microfiber cloth, and then spray hydrogen peroxide and wipe that off.

Insect repellent

- Mix equal parts water and vinegar in a quart spray bottle

- Add 20 drops peppermint essential oil

Spray around door to repel spiders, cockroaches, and ants.

Remove Tea and Coffee Stains from your clothes

- 1 Tbsp warm water

- 1 Tbsp white vinegar

- 1 Tbsp laundry detergent.

Mix ingredients together and apply it to your stain. It works great!

Odor and Stain Remover

You can use vinegar to clean the stains and odors from plastic food containers, lunch boxes, plastic toys, and other items. Spray them with a generous amount of vinegar, let them sit for two minutes and then wipe them clean with a microfiber cloth.

Clean the Toilet

Pour a cup of white vinegar into the toilet and let it sit for several hours or overnight to remove hard water stains. It will also clean the bowl. Swish with a toilet brush before flushing.

Shiny Faucets

Spray your faucets with vinegar and then wipe them with a microfiber cloth. For old faucets use the Vinegar Scouring Paste.

Vinegar Scouring Paste

- 2 Tbsp vinegar

- 4 Tbsp sea salt

- 5 drops essential oils

Mix these together and use an old toothbrush or rag to clean old faucets and get them looking new again. To clean the BBQ grill, spray the grate with distilled white vinegar, then scrub it with a wire brush.

Clean Shower Heads

Clean the showerheads by placing 1 cup of vinegar in a plastic sandwich bag. Place the bag of vinegar solution over the showerhead and secure it in place with tape. Leave overnight, then remove it and scrub clean. It will get rid of the lime build up.

Shower, Tub and Tile cleaner

- 2 cups white vinegar

- 2 Tbsp dish soap

- 15 drops lemon essential oil (or your preference)

Put everything in a spray bottle and clean away! The dish soap will help get rid of the greasy soap scum whilst the vinegar will clean and sanitize and the essential oils will smell amazing(they also have their own antibacterial properties as well, depending on which oil you use)

Clean Leather Handbags, Chairs and Shoes

Get a vinegar-soaked microfiber cloth and you can wipe down

your shoes, handbags, leather couches and chairs.

Clean the Microwave

Use equal parts vinegar and water and pour into a bowl. Heat in the microwave for a few minutes and leave the bowl sitting in there for a few more minutes. Remove the bowl with oven mitts as it may be hot and wipe the microwave clean!

Clean the Coffee Maker

Reduce hard water buildup and disinfect the coffee pot at the same time by cleaning the coffee pot with vinegar. Drain all water from the system, then fill it with vinegar and run a full cycle. Follow the vinegar wash with a rinse water cycle before making coffee again. Do this every couple of months.

Clean your Computer Screen

Shut down computer and use equal parts vinegar and distilled water in a spray bottle. Do not spray directly onto the screen. Spray onto your microfiber cloth and then wipe your screen.

Window Cleaner

- 1 cup distilled water

- 1 cup vinegar

- 1 Tbsp dish soap (if the windows are greasy)

- 10 drops peppermint essential oil

Pour everything into a spray bottle and use.

Wood Ring Cleaner Recipe

- 1 Tbsp vinegar

- 1 Tbsp olive oil

Mix everything in a bowl and use to get rid of those white rings on your furniture. Rub the rings in the direction of the wood grain. When you have them rubbed out, buff the surface with a microfiber cloth.

Wood Furniture Polish 1

- 1 Tbsp Olive Oil

- 1/4 cup White Vinegar

- 10 drops Lemon essential oil

- 10 drops Cedarwood essential oil

- 5 drops Orange essential oil

- 4-ounce Spray Bottle

Mix all ingredients and shake before use. Spray and wipe.

Get Rid of Food Odors in The Kitchen

If you have a smelly kitchen from cooking fish for example, simmer 1 cup of white vinegar in a pot and bring it to a boil. Let it simmer on the stove until most of the liquid has evaporated. Your kitchen may smell of vinegar for a while, but it will remove the fishy smell.

Clean Stainless-Steel Appliances

Spray vinegar onto your stainless steel and wipe off with a microfiber cloth.

Kitchen Degreaser Spray

- 1 cup distilled water

- 1 cup vinegar

- 1 Tbsp dish soap

- 10 drops lemon essential oil

Pour all ingredients in a spray bottle.

Deodorize Lunch Boxes and Plastic Containers

Spray them with vinegar and wipe clean

Disinfect your Cutting Boards

Wash the cutting board front and back with hot soapy water, rinse it, and dry. Spray with vinegar and then wipe off.

Make Your Dishes Shine

Put 1/4 cup of white vinegar into your dishwasher's final rinse. It removes water spots and rinses away all the soap residue.

Fabric Softener

Add ¼ cup of white vinegar to the fabric softener dispenser on your washing machine or just put it in the rinse cycle.

Fruit and Vegetable Wash

Mix up a 50/50 vinegar/water solution to use for washing fresh fruits and vegetables. The vinegar dissolves wax that may be coating the surface and removes pesticide residues. Rinse the vegetables and fruits thoroughly with water.

Clean Garden and Patio Furniture

White vinegar is the base of a simple homemade all-purpose cleaner to wipe all your metal and plastic garden and patio furniture.

Flower Preserving Recipe

Add 1 Tbsp vinegar and 1 Tbsp sugar to your vase water to make your flowers last longer. It also gives them new life if they are starting to droop.

Remove Ink Marks

Spray vinegar onto ink mark, then scrub the spot until all the ink is gone

Clean and Disinfect the Refrigerator

Use a solution of half white vinegar and half water to clean the interior of the fridge. A quick spray and wipe down will remove odors, clean the interior, and kills off mildew and mold spores as well as germs that might be lurking.

Clean the Toilet

Pour a cup of white vinegar into the toilet and let it sit for several hours or overnight. It dissolves hard water stains and cleans the bowl. Scrub the toilet with a toilet brush before flushing.

Remove Antiperspirant Stains

White vinegar gently removes stains on clothing caused by antiperspirants and even light scorch marks from ironing. Apply white vinegar on a soft cloth and gently rub the stain.

Remove Old Paint from Brushes

Place paint brushes in a pot of vinegar and let them soak for an hour or more. Then turn the stove on and bring the vinegar to a simmer. Drain the vinegar and rinse the brushes clean.

Scouring Paste

- 1 teaspoon of white vinegar

- 2 tablespoons of table salt

- 10 drops essential oil

This is great whenever you need to do some scouring!

Shiny Faucets

Clean your faucets with vinegar. Give them a spray and allow to soak for a minute before buffing them clean with a soft cloth.

Eliminate Litter Box Odors

Remove unwelcome litter box odor by cleaning it with distilled white vinegar. Empty the litter box and add 1/2 inch of vinegar to cover the bottom. Let it stand for a half hour, then rinse it with cold water.

Erase Crayon from Walls and Floor

Crayons are made of wax and will dissolve in white vinegar. Use a small brush dipped in vinegar to scrub the crayon marks, then wipe the stains away with a microfiber cloth.

Remove Odors on Fabrics, Carpets, and Furniture

Spray your furniture, carpets, dog beds, and other fabrics with a fine mist of distilled white vinegar. The vinegar neutralizes odors and freshens up the room.

Clean Dishwasher

Remove soap and food residues in the dishwasher by pouring a cup of vinegar into the empty dishwasher and running it through a full cycle. Repeat this once a month to keep your dishwasher clean, reduce hard water buildup, and disinfect it.

Clean a Mattress or Upholstery

- 1/4 cup Laundry detergent

- 1/4 cup vinegar

- 2 cups of water

- 10 drops essential oils

Put the ingredients into a spray bottle and spray cleaner very lightly on the mattress and let it sit for half an hour. Then use a towel and blot the area until all food stains are gone. After vacuuming the mattress will be clean and stain free.

Mineral Deposits on Steam Iron

- 1 cup distilled water

- 1 cup vinegar

Mix these together and fill up your steam iron. Using this mixture in the steaming position will free up any clogged holes and clean the base plate of the iron naturally.

Revitalize Leather Furniture

- 1/2 cup vinegar

- 1/2 cup linseed oil

- 10 drops essential oil

Put all ingredients into a spray bottle and spray on then buff with a microfiber cloth. Do a spot test first to be sure.

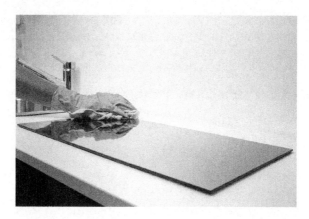

Hydrogen Peroxide Uses

What Is Hydrogen Peroxide? It is the only germicidal agent that consists of only oxygen and water. It kills disease organisms through the process of oxidation, and it is thought to be the world's safest, all-natural sanitizer!

You want to use the 3% hydrogen peroxide. Hydrogen peroxide is nontoxic and considered extremely safe however if you have a skin reaction discontinue use. Please consult your doctor if you are unsure of use.

The U.S. Environmental Protection Agency has approved hydrogen peroxide as a sanitizer! Below are some great recipes for Hydrogen Peroxide:

Disinfect Small Wounds

Hydrogen peroxide is a natural antiseptic, therefore one of its most common uses is to clean wounds to prevent infection.

Prevent "Swimmer's Ear"

Mix equal parts hydrogen peroxide and vinegar in a small dropper bottle. Put several drops in each ear after swimming to prevent infection.

Relieve Ear Infections

Put 6-8 drops in the ear, then rest the opposite side of the head downward. After about five minutes, turn the head over and let the excess run back out into a tissue or cotton ball. You can do this 4 times per day to resolve an infection. Consult a doctor before trying though, especially on children.

Remove Ear Wax

Put a couple of drops of hydrogen peroxide into ears, wait a minute or two, then follow up with a couple of drops of olive oil. Wait another minute, then drain fluid from ears to remove ear wax.

Oral Rinse for Teeth Whitening and Bad Breath

Use a cap full of hydrogen peroxide as a mouth rinse to help whiten teeth and kill germs that cause bad breath.

Disinfect Toothbrushes

Soak toothbrushes in hydrogen peroxide to disinfect them and remove bacteria.

Whiten Your Nails

Soak fingertips and toes in hydrogen peroxide to naturally whiten your nails.

Acne Treatment

Use hydrogen peroxide as a face rinse to kill the bacteria that cause acne and help clear your complexion. You could also dab with a cotton ball

Soften Corns & Calluses

Mix equal parts hydrogen peroxide and warm water to make a foot soak that will naturally soften corns and calluses.

Treat Foot Fungus

Combine equal parts hydrogen peroxide and water and apply to affected skin each day

Clean Tile Surfaces

Spray hydrogen peroxide directly onto tile to remove dirt and stains.

Whiten Grout

Spray onto your grout and then leave for about an hour or so and then wipe off with a damp cloth

Remove Stains and Clean Toilet and Bathtub

Pour half a cup of hydrogen peroxide into your toilet bowl or tub and leave it for 30 minutes. Scrub clean.

Mold & Mildew

Spray hydrogen peroxide on mold and mildew to stop fungal growth.

Window/Mirror cleaner

Spray hydrogen peroxide on dirty mirrors and other glass surfaces and then wipe off.

Disinfect Countertops

Spray hydrogen peroxide on kitchen and bathroom countertops to clean and disinfect.

Soak Sponges to Disinfect and Remove Smells

Soak sponges in hydrogen peroxide for 15 – 30 minutes.

Wash Fruits & Vegetables

Spray fruits and veggies and then leave for a minute. Rinse with clean water to remove dirt, wax, etc.

Disinfect Cutting Boards

Spray hydrogen peroxide on cutting boards to kill germs and bacteria especially from foods such as raw meat.

Pot Cleaner

Mix Hydrogen Peroxide with some baking soda to form a paste and rub it onto baked on foods and let it sit for several minutes. Then scrub clean.

Refrigerator cleaner

Spray the inside of your refrigerator and leave for a few minutes. Wipe clean for a clean disinfected fridge surface.

Whiten Laundry

Add about a cup of hydrogen peroxide to your wash cycle but be careful as it acts as a bleach. Only use it with whites, not colored fabric.

Stain remover

Mix hydrogen peroxide with liquid castile soap to make a paste and apply to stains (coffee, wine, blood, sweat, etc.) to remove them. Remember, hydrogen peroxide will bleach darker fabrics. Use this technique with caution!

Clean Rugs & Carpets

Spray hydrogen peroxide onto light-colored carpets and rugs to remove stains from mud, food, etc. Just remember that hydrogen peroxide will bleach some fabrics. Do a small test on an area.

Refresh Re-useable Bags

Spray hydrogen peroxide inside your re-useable cloth shopping bags to clean, disinfect, and remove food odors.

Disinfect Lunchboxes

Spray hydrogen peroxide into lunchboxes and coolers

Seed Germination

Improve Seed Germination. Soak seeds in 1 tsp of hydrogen peroxide and 1 cup of water solution to remove fungal spores and help seeds germinate more quickly.

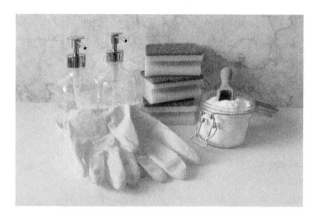

Baking Soda Uses

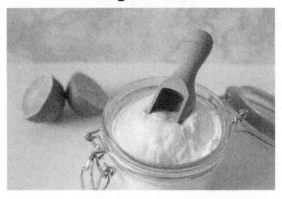

Who knew there were so many uses for baking soda other than baking and removing odors in your fridge? Listed below you will find many fabulous recipes including cleaning your bathtub, oven, microwave and more!

Scrubbing Paste

- 1 cup baking soda

- 3 tbsp castile soap

- 1 tbsp cornstarch

- 1 tbsp white vinegar

- 15 drops Lemon (Citrus limon)

- 15 drops Tea Tree (Melaleuca alternifolia)

Mix all your ingredients and essential oils together in the wide mouth container. Add more castile soap as needed to make a smooth consistency. Use about a teaspoon of this mixture on a sponge to clean the shower, and the kitchen and bathroom sinks.

Bathtub Cleaner

Sprinkle baking soda around tub. Wet sponge and apply a few drops of dawn dishwashing soap and clean tub.

Stainless Steel Sink Cleaner

Sprinkle baking soda around sink and use a damp sponge to clean sink.

Stovetops

Sprinkle baking soda on stove top and spray hot water to absorb soda. Let sit for approximately 30 minutes and scrub clean.

Microwave

Put 3 Tbsp of baking soda in a bowl of water and place in microwave. Heat for 3 – 5 minutes. When microwave stops, keep the door closed to give the moisture and steam the heated bowl of water generated to have time to work. Remove bowl with oven mitt or towel and take a moist, warm sponge to the wipe the inside of the microwave.

Roasting Pans

Sprinkle pan with baking soda, pour hot water over top about an inch or two deep and soak for one hour. For stubborn build up, you can boil it first with baking soda in the pot.

Dishwasher

Freshen things up by sprinkling a layer of bicarb on the bottom of the dishwasher. Close it and let it sit overnight. The next day take a damp sponge and scrub the powder into the inside walls and door of the dishwasher. Remove most of the powder then run a full cycle on empty to remove all traces of the powder.

Another method to freshen up the dishwasher is to toss in a cup of baking soda to an empty dishwasher then run it on the rinse cycle.

Refrigerator Freshener

After cleaning the refrigerator, keep it smelling fresh with an open box of baking soda.

Coffee Mug Stains

Remove stains from coffee mugs by wiping mug with a wet cloth then rub the inside of the mug with soda. If the stains are stubborn, soak overnight in hot water and baking soda.

Thermos Cleaner

Put 1 Tbsp of baking soda in thermos bottle, fill with boiling water and then leave the cap closed for a few hours and rinse.

Air Freshener Spray

Mix 1 cup hot water with 1 Tbsp baking soda and 15 drops of your favorite essential oils. Shake to dissolve and spray wherever in the house you need it.

Carpet Freshener

Sprinkle carpets with baking soda and leave for 2 hours and vacuum.

Floor Scuff & Stain Remover

Mix with water to make a paste, apply to wet sponge, and scrub out the scuff marks.

Tile Grout

Make a paste of baking soda and water. Use to scrub grout clean with a sponge, leave for a few minutes, then rinse clean.

Goo Remover

Mix baking soda and coconut oil to make a paste then rub gently into the goo, then wipe off with a warm wet cloth.

Grease Stain on Garage Floor

Sprinkle on the stain and scrub off with water.

Fishy Smell

Fish or onion smells can be removed from plates, pots, pans etc. by adding 1 Tbsp of baking soda to the dish water.

Suitcase/Backpack Freshener

If your suitcase or backpack have not been used for a while and have a musty smell, they can be freshened up by sprinkling baking soda inside, then close the case and then let sit a day or two. Vacuum the baking soda out.

Musty Books

For books that are musty, sprinkle baking soda on the pages and allow time to air out. If there's mildew on the paper, you can rub the soda into the spots and lay out to bleach in the sun.

Crayon Marks on Wall

Make a paste with baking soda and water then use it to gently scrub the marks.

Mattress Refresher

Sprinkle onto your mattresses, leave for an hour or two and then vacuum up.

Laundry Booster

Add ½ Cup of baking soda to a load of wash.

Preventing Deodorant Stains on your Clothes

Apply baking soda to your underarms after applying deodorant.

Bad Breath

Rinse with a solution of water and baking soda.

Teeth whitener

Mix baking soda with coconut oil and brush your teeth.

Sunburn Relief

Add a cup of baking soda to a bath.

Insect Repellent

Mix equal parts white sugar and baking soda to kill ants, cockroaches, etc.

Bite and Sting Relief

Mix a paste with water and apply.

Foaming Hand Cleanser

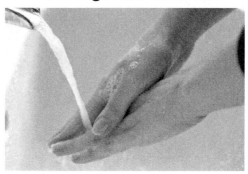

Making your own hand soap is super easy! In the recipe below you can use your preference of essential oils or carrier oil.

- 2 tbsp Castile Soap

- ½ to 1 tsp of Sweet Almond Oil

- 10 – 15 drops of lemon essential oil (can use more or less depending upon preference of scent)

- 8 oz PET bottle or glass bottle with foaming pump top

Fill the bottle with Castile soap and essential oils. Fill the rest with water about ¼ from the top of bottle.

Toilet Bowl Bombs

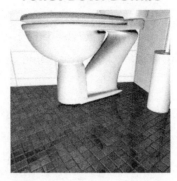

Clean your toilet naturally without harmful chemicals! Just drop one in your toilet boil, watch it fizz, dissolve, and swish your toilet brush around the bowl to clean!

- 1 cup of baking soda

- 1/4 cup of citric acid

- 20-30 drops of essential oil

- Spray bottle with water, distilled water, or hydrogen peroxide

- Round tin molds or ice trey

Mix all the dry ingredients in a large bowl. Add the essential oils and mix. Spray the mixture with water or witch hazel until you get a "wet sand" consistency. Mixture should not crumble in your hands. (Use gloves if you have sensitive skin.)

Press the mixture into the molds and let sit for 24 to 48 hours to harden. Store in an airtight container.

If you are using the round metal molds, over-fill each half of the mold with mixture and then press the two halves together. Wipe off excess mixture on the outside and gently pull apart and place round bomb in hand and place on wax paper or aluminum foil to harden for 24hrs. Store in an airtight container. (Tip: If the mixture falls apart when you take the bomb out of the mold, it's not wet enough. Place back into the bowl and spritz with more witch hazel or water.)

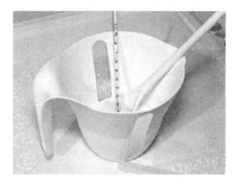

Conclusion

"The health of the people is really the foundation upon which all their happiness and all their powers as a state depend."

-Benjamin Disraeli

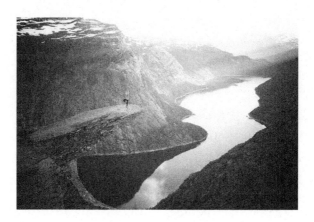

References

Perron-Jones, M. (2019, November 9). Aromatherapy- Using Essential Oils For Natural Living- Retrieved from http://www.udemy.com/course/aromatherapy-how-to-use-essential-oils-in-your-everyday-life/

Salvo, S. (2007). Massage Therapy: Principles and Practice. St Louis, MS: Saunders Elsevier

ABOUT THE AUTHOR

Jennifer Spivey is an Aromatherapy Practitioner, Licensed Massage Therapist, and Reiki Master/Practitioner who resides in Bluffton, SC with her beagle mix, "Luna." She was introduced to Aromatherapy when she began a career in massage therapy and has been obsessed with these magical oils ever since. Being a huge advocate of spiritual and holistic healing herself, she wanted to share what she has learned over the years with others in hopes they will benefit from these precious oils as she has.

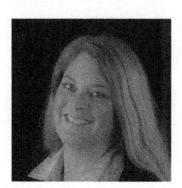

Can You Help?

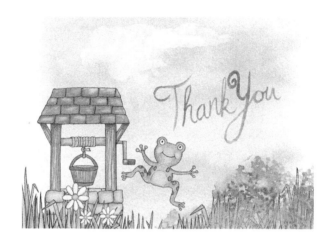

Thanks So Much For Reading My Book!

I really appreciate your feedback, and I love hearing what you have to say.

I need your input to make the next version of this book and my future books better.

Please leave an honest review on Amazon letting me know what you thought of the book.

Index

Printed in Great Britain
by Amazon

28701789R00099